PUBLIC HEALTH SPATIAL PLANNING IN PRACTICE

Improving Health and Wellbeing

Michael Chao-Jung Chang, Liz Green
and Carl Petrokofsky

P

First published in Great Britain in 2022 by

Policy Press, an imprint of
Bristol University Press
University of Bristol
1–9 Old Park Hill
Bristol
BS2 8BB
UK
t: +44 (0)117 374 6645
e: bup-info@bristol.ac.uk

Details of international sales and distribution partners are available at
policy.bristoluniversitypress.co.uk

© Bristol University Press 2022

British Library Cataloguing in Publication Data
A catalogue record for this book is available from the British Library

ISBN 978-1-4473-5846-6 paperback
ISBN 978-1-4473-5847-3 ePub
ISBN 978-1-4473-5848-0 ePdf

The right of Michael Chao-Jung Chang, Liz Green and Carl Petrokofsky to be
identified as authors of this work has been asserted by them in accordance with the
Copyright, Designs and Patents Act 1988.

All rights reserved: no part of this publication may be reproduced, stored in a
retrieval system or transmitted in any form or by any means, electronic, mechanical,
photocopying, recording or otherwise, without the prior permission of Bristol
University Press.

Every reasonable effort has been made to obtain permission to reproduce copyrighted
material. If, however, anyone knows of an oversight, please contact the publisher.

The statements and opinions contained within this publication are solely those of
the authors and not of the University of Bristol or Bristol University Press. The
University of Bristol and Bristol University Press disclaim responsibility for any injury
to persons or property resulting from any material published in this publication.

Bristol University Press and Policy Press work to counter discrimination on grounds
of gender, race, disability, age and sexuality.

Cover design: Andrew Corbett
Front cover image: Berkeley Homes
Bristol University Press and Policy Press use environmentally
responsible print partners.
Printed and bound in Great Britain by CMP, Poole

Contents

List of figures and tables

Figures

Tables

List of insider stories

List of abbreviations

CPD	continuing professional development
EIA	environmental impact assessment
HIA	Health Impact Assessment
HiAP	Health in All Policies
MHCLG	Ministry of Housing, Communities and Local Government (now Department for Levelling Up, Housing and Communities)
NCD	non-communicable diseases
NHS	National Health Service
NPPF	National Planning Policy Framework
PHE	Public Health England (PHE was abolished on 1 October 2021 and its functions moved to the UK Health Security Agency and the Office for Health Improvement and Disparities)
RTPI	Royal Town Planning Institute
SEA	strategic environmental assessment
TCPA	Town and Country Planning Association
WHIASU	Wales Health Impact Assessment Support Unit
WHO	World Health Organization

Glossary

built environment The spaces, places and land uses, including buildings and infrastructure that make up the fabric of the environment that people and society use and require to function and thrive.

epidemiology The study of the cause and distribution of disease or health states in populations. It is the science that underpins public health and is concerned with: diagnosis or health event (what); person (who); place (where); time (when); and causes, risk factors and modes of transmission (why/how).

health inequalities or disparities Differences in health status or in the distribution of wider determinants of health between different population groups and geographical areas.

health and wellbeing A state of physical, mental and social wellbeing. It implies physical and mental health and can only be achieved by addressing the range of socio-economic, biological and environmental factors that impact on individuals and communities. In this book, the term 'health and wellbeing' indicates parity of importance between physical and mental health and social wellbeing.

planning (spatial and land use) Processes and structures that shape the design, consenting decisions and management of the built environment, and ensure the right development happens in the right place at the right time, benefitting current and future communities.

practitioners Anyone engaged and working in planning and public health, as well as in policy creation, land use development, urban design, commissioning, lobbying and advocacy, and decision-making.

public health The science and art of preventing disease, prolonging life and promoting health and wellbeing.

wider determinants of health The causes of the causes, such as the social, economic and environmental conditions that influence the health and wellbeing of individuals and populations.

Acknowledgements

This book contains a collection of knowledge, insight, experiences and research developed over the years from pioneering and committed practitioners and academicians. The authors acknowledge their contribution in a morally charged agenda that is deserving of more formal recognition in regulatory, professional and career-development pathways, and hope that this book makes a useful contribution to the cause.

The authors thank all those practitioners who provided insight through the 'insider stories' and sharing their experiences of day-to-day practices. We know there are many others who will be able to share their experiences, and there will be many good practices we can highlight. Therefore, we collectively celebrate their efforts and actions, successes and failures, as we work towards a shared goal of mainstreaming the policy and practice of planning for health.

On a personal level, the authors are grateful for the support of loved ones, family, friends and colleagues through the journey of research and writing the book. We would especially like to thank John, Susan and Rachel Green, Lee Parry-Williams, Dr Andrew Buroni, Martin Seymour, Dr Flora Ogilvie, Dr Gillian Petrokofsky, and Max Petrokofsky for their critical analysis and help in specific chapters. Their timely encouragement and support have been invaluable.

The authors thank Katy Cooper for her editing of the book and Policy Press for providing a platform for the authors to reach a wider practitioner audience through the publication of this book.

Introduction

> Working together, planning and public health
> professionals can ensure that health promotion,
> disease prevention and better health equity through
> good UTP [urban and territorial planning] is a central
> component of communicable and noncommunicable
> disease reduction and management responses.
>
> UN-Habitat and World Health
> Organization (2020)

There is a professional paradigm shift taking place. Across built environment and public health professions and sectors, practitioners are rediscovering their role in shaping what matters to people and their relationship with the environment in terms of mental and physical health and wellbeing. Increasingly, there is an emergence and embedding of such terms as 'health', 'wellbeing', 'wellness', 'public health' and 'health inequalities' into the legal and professional languages of those involved in and tasked with shaping, creating and investing in places and spaces. In turn, strategies designed by these practitioners to improve health and wellbeing are making reference to the built and natural environment as fundamental to addressing and preventing the causes of ill health, and promoting better health.

Spatial planning for public health is a positive and exciting new interdisciplinary area of practice. The opportunities, possibilities and potential of this approach have been recognised in policy and practice, and, in many areas, have begun to develop dedicated workforce resources. The authors are motivated by the fact that practitioners are actively seeking advice, support and the confidence regarding how to more effectively implement the knowledge, evidence and skills they possess. There is a distinct need for a text that can clearly articulate how the spatial, planning and health agendas can come together to mobilise policies, plans and actions to support healthy places and communities. Arguably, the concept of improving people's quality of life was never lost in the modus operandi of those professions. The professional history and roots of built environment professions, such as architects, planners and urban designers, are deeply embedded in public health, with the foundations of Garden Cities in Letchworth in England then spreading worldwide being a prime example. Likewise, the origins of public health lie in sanitation and engineering solutions to address severe disease outbreaks in industrial urban areas. However, somehow, the role that the built and natural environment played in shaping healthy behaviours was, if not lost, certainly not at the forefront of the work of these professionals.

Recent research has identified barriers and challenges to effective spatial planning for public health. For example, there has been a lack of clarity in determining those aspects of people's quality of life that we are protecting and improving through legislation, policy and evidence. Professional understanding of quality of life has evolved over time from a health protection approach, such as through improving water quality to prevent a series of communicable diseases, into a multifaceted approach that seeks to tackle the root causes of ill health by addressing the contribution arising directly from our built environment or how it shapes our behaviours. It has taken the explicit involvement of the public health and wider health professions in the discourse to see a marked transformation in how planning and planners approach land-use planning.

There has been a growing appreciation by professionals of how the built and natural environment, as well as the socio-economic environments in which people live, play a role equal to, or more important than, healthcare services in helping people to maintain health and wellbeing. Evidence has shown that people's socio-economic and physical environment is a significant determinant of 60 per cent of their health status, while the healthcare system and individual genetics account for 25 per cent and 15 per cent, respectively. While the proportions may vary from place to place, country to country, the overarching premise is that to keep people healthy, at least equal attention must be paid to improving the environment and conditions in which people live as to improving the health and care system. While spatial planning may have contributed to poor-quality environments and health outcomes in the past, there is a real recognition today that it is a key delivery tool for protecting, maintaining and improving population health.

There has been improvement in the state of practices in planning for health: international frameworks, such as the United Nations (UN) Sustainable Development Goals (SDGs), are seeking tangible actions to both improve health and wellbeing and to reduce inequalities as cultural, economic, governmental and professional norms. National planning strategies have begun to emphasise the social role of planning towards supporting the development of healthy and equitable communities on a par with the achievement of other socio-economic, environmental and sustainability objectives. At a local level, planning policy practice has also begun to orient towards actions designed to address specific health and wellbeing needs of communities. While practice may not have been mainstreamed yet, there are encouraging signs of a greater reuniting of health with planning in many localities and countries.

Definition of public health spatial planning in practice

Public health spatial planning in practice is the process of practitioners from any profession working within and across respective systems, structures and policy areas related to the built and natural environment committing to advance the practice of planning for health. It requires an understanding of and working competency in the art, planning law, political and social sciences to implement effective actions with a primary directive to improve public health outcomes and reduce health inequalities for all individuals, communities and places.

Public health spatial planning propositions

There are three propositions on the practice of public health spatial planning to put forward to readers, which form the overarching narrative of this book.

The built and natural environment matters to health

Poor health not only affects the welfare of individuals and their families, but also has ripple effects that impact on local neighbourhoods and communities, and ultimately on wider society and national and local economies. Fundamental flaws in the planning and design of the built and natural environment can exacerbate disparities in health between individuals and communities. On the other hand, sensitive design of the built and natural environment can ameliorate or even prevent much ill health. The effect can be profound for those individuals and communities who are most vulnerable and at risk, and have fewer options and opportunities to influence matters outside their control. These are the people and communities who will be disproportionately disadvantaged by a poor environment; hence, a focus on a well-designed, health-promoting physical environment becomes a matter of social justice. The financial gain arising from improved community wellbeing to wider society, national and local economies, and health systems can be substantial, and has been shown to outweigh the costs of inaction.

Planning matters to health

Planning is a critical tool used by national and local governments as well as communities. Planners and other built environment professionals play a pivotal role in making decisions about the environment that will last generations. The emerging consensus about how the environment shapes people's health and wellbeing can be related to: the location, type and quality of homes provided; the amount of green space available for leisure; or the safety and security of the streets that pedestrians and cyclists use. The planning system, its legislative frameworks and its interconnection with urban development dynamics describe those principles that are prioritised in practice and how decisions based on these are made that shape our environment. Effective and proactive planning practices for health matter. Planning for health does not happen by default. Having a strong, health-oriented regulatory framework is necessary to ensure due process and achieve outcomes. Integrating public health into the planning system can help to institutionalise wellbeing considerations into the legal and professional psyche. The emergence of tools to help address health and wellbeing issues, such as Health Impact Assessments (HIAs) and evidence-based planning for health frameworks, and engagement processes with stakeholders enables planners and the planning system to address and consider local health challenges, and to stay relevant to the communities they serve. Such integration can help reframe the purpose of planning beyond a mechanistic regulatory and land-allocation tool into one that helps it to achieve its original aspirations for quality of life and quality of place for people.

The professional workforce matters to health

The role of public health practitioners is critical to providing a coherent professional voice on the impacts of the design of our towns and cities on health and wellbeing. Their role also provides both a spearhead and a bridge to their local communities to ascertain and identify health needs, and to communicate these to those responsible for addressing such matters through design and planning, be they planners or local elected officials taking final decisions on land-use policy.

The role of planning practitioners is critical in ensuring that health is built into all planning decisions at both the policy level and the earliest possible stages of a project design and development. A range of professions, including town and urban planners, architects, landscape architects, transport planners, and urban designers, are the purveyors of public health. They must realise the crucial importance of their work to building, maintaining and protecting the public's health.

Many practitioners are breaking new ground – or rediscovering their public health/planning roots – with the emergence of a new cadre of integrated planning and health practitioners with shared competencies and knowledge. An early pioneer was Dr Norman Macfadyen, a local doctor who was the medical officer of health of Letchworth Garden City in England. From 1929 to 1944, he was the chairman of the executive committee of what later became the Town and Country Planning Association (TCPA) – Britain's oldest charity concerned with planning, housing and the environment. Recent pioneers include those with joint degrees in planning and public health, and those planning and/or public health practitioners with a dedicated local government role as 'public health spatial planners'.

Book structure overview

This book has been structured to provide a consistent narrative with, evidence leading to improving the art and science of public health spatial planning practice and action (see Figure I.1). It draws on a range of UK and international sources and experiences:

- Part I provides an overview of spatial planning's important contribution to preventing disease, promoting, maintaining and improving health, and reducing health inequalities. By acknowledging the evidence, this section makes the case for planning and health, and then considers aspects of the policies and professionals to make this happen, with an overview of the current state of play.
- Part II highlights specific planning powers and approaches to achieve public health outcomes, as well as their brief history and application. These include a Health in All Policies (HiAP) approach, HIAs and other regulatory tools. It illustrates these powers from the UK context but also highlights comparisons and applicability across other countries.
- Part III describes the state of integration of public health and spatial planning, and the potential implications of various research, initiatives and actions for achieving national and local public health outcomes.
- Part IV identifies and makes the value-added case for healthy urban development projects. It will help demonstrate the

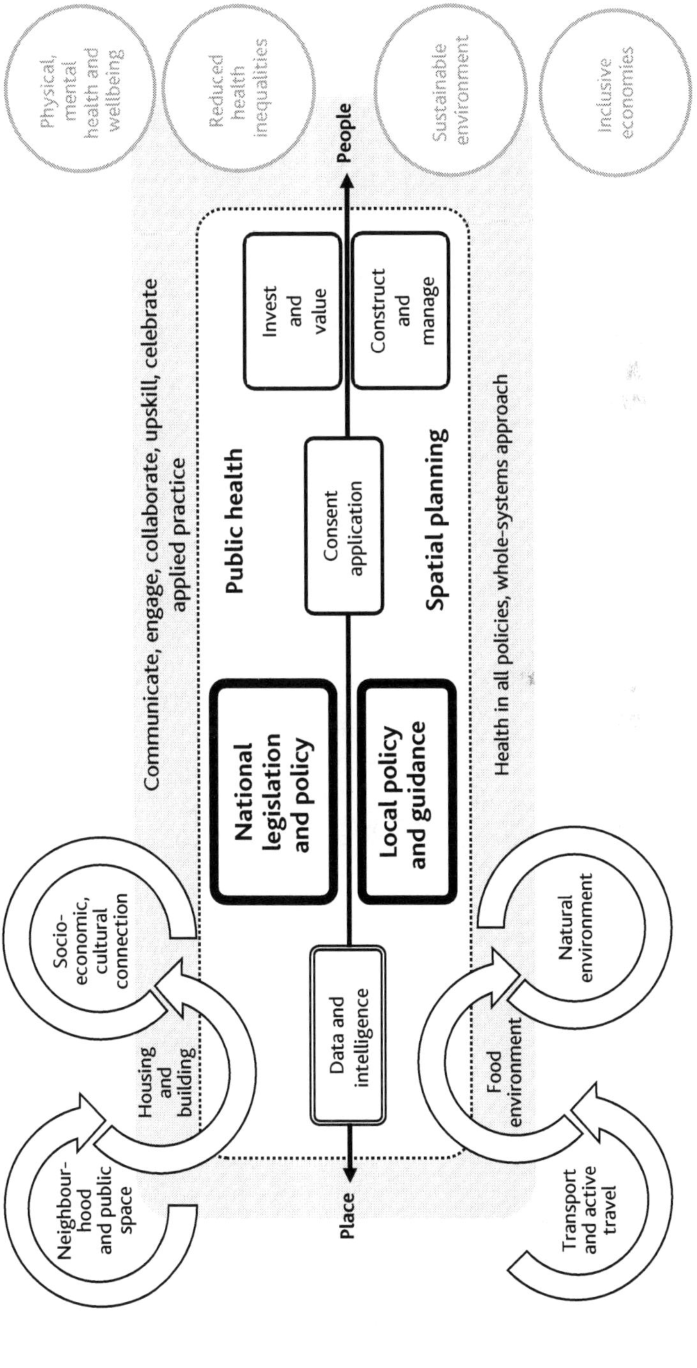

Figure I.1: Art and science of public health spatial planning in practice

multiple beneficiaries of healthy planning, from social value to improvement in property premiums, and how practices have evolved in public–private partnerships.

- Part V finally frames the basis for future action by recognising the post-COVID-19 pandemic reality to scan the horizon for some emerging issues/trends/system changes that could have a positive or adverse impact on the existing state of practice of public health spatial planning.

Interspersed throughout the chapters are 'insider stories'. These are contributions from practitioners that provide insider perspectives on a specific element of public health spatial planning practice in a locality or a profession, and how such practices have sought to improve public health through planning.

Audience groups

The target audience for this book will be wide ranging, but the emphasis is on building the knowledge, skills and competency of those professionals involved in creating, planning, delivering and researching how healthy environments can be developed through sensitive spatial planning. We hope that all readers will gain a baseline knowledge on how to work together more effectively to create 'healthy places' in order to be better armed to engage more effectively with the planning system to achieve local priorities.

The book aims to provide clarity around certain questions for readers with the following backgrounds and interests:

- *For public health professionals* and policymakers with wider determinants portfolios: where are the key windows of opportunity through the planning process and what actions could be undertaken?
- *For spatial planners* working across all stages of the system: how can the planning system and processes improve your recognition and consideration of health, and deliver outcomes?
- *For urban development project delivery partners*: what are your contributions, and how can health issues be embedded in your planning and investment approaches?

- *For wider built and natural environment professionals* (in housing, transport, environmental health and urban design): how can your complementary roles and contributions be better recognised and utilised during the planning processes?
- *For academics and research centres* on healthy environments, built environment, property, public health and health policy: in what ways can your research form a more practical and relevant evidence base for planning policies and decisions?
- *For healthcare commissioners and providers*: how can a better understanding of upstream prevention actions benefit you in terms of reduced pressures on services while leveraging value from urban development to improve health and care infrastructure services in the community?
- *For educators and students of the aforementioned disciplines and professions*: how can you ensure that learning and development better reflect and meet the needs of professionals in the workplace, and recognise the exciting range of options for career selection and development?

COVID-19 implications

We cannot write a book about planning for health in this pathbreaking period of human history without acknowledging and cross-referencing COVID-19 and its impacts. The writing for this book started at the height of COVID-19. It has taken a pandemic to galvanise consensus on healthy environments across professions, industries and sectors. A pandemic serves as a teachable reminder of the effect that the built environment has on people's exposure to infectious disease and on their physical and mental wellbeing. The book concludes with a final chapter that looks ahead at the ripple effect of the pandemic and other trends and signals on the practice of public health spatial planning.

Concluding statement

Using the planning system to improve public health may feel like trying to 'fit a square peg into a round hole' scenario. This feeling is understandable, as the planning system already exists to address a multiplicity of social, economic and environmental issues and needs. This book will help prepare practitioners for the journey ahead, as the gains to be made in improved health and wellbeing for our communities are so great.

This book will not only support practitioners in better understanding how best to use existing planning tools, but also introduce other tools specific to achieving public health outcomes. Using the authors' combined experiences and expertise, the book aims to instil confidence in those public health spatial planners with responsibilities, directly or indirectly, for improving people's health and wellbeing. We look forward to continuing conversations with practitioners to improve and celebrate the art and science of the practice of public health spatial planning.

Pre-reading reflection: having picked up this book, put it down and step outside!

Ramble observantly down your lane, neighbourhood, town or city, and carefully note the buildings, roads, parks and pavements. How are people using these spaces individually and in groups, and how is the design of those same buildings, roads, parks and pavements influencing their behaviours – and yours?

Does the street environment inspire you to take a walk or cycle around the neighbourhood? Are children able to get outside and run around in the park or walk or cycle to school in safe circumstances? Are people with limited mobility able to access the same services as everyone else, or are there impediments in the built environment that have been designed without regard to the needs of the whole community in mind? Can you buy fresh fruit and vegetables locally, or do you live in a 'food desert' with no nearby access to healthier food options to encourage a healthy diet? Do the traffic congestion, noise, lack of pleasant surroundings and walkable spaces, and poorly managed public spaces make you think again about enjoying your local neighbourhood?

Welcome back! Now, having come back inside with your eyes, ears and senses freshly attuned to your surroundings, are you filled with feelings of tranquillity and peacefulness, invigorated by a walk in the fresh air in a park surrounded by greenery and water features? Or, rather, are you feeling alert, on edge, stressed and overly stimulated due to a sensory onslaught spent dodging overbearing traffic, noise, smells or smog?

Are you still asking: what does any of this have to do with health? This book is about how professionals can influence the impact of the quality and design of the environment on health and wellbeing. All too often, we find that the built environment actually makes it more difficult to choose the conditions that are known to sustain good health, and we need to reflect on our role and responsibility as professionals.

PART I

Scene setting

Working together to create healthier environments will not happen by magic. People who are making progress on this have an excellent understanding of the purpose of planning and the role of evidence. They look methodically for the hooks that matter locally, build networks, stay up to date with policy and practice, and work within corporate systems and processes to make a case for change as and when they can.

Chang and Ross (2012, p 37)

The factors impacting on people's health and wellbeing are complex, and can be broadly described as relating to an individual's genetic inheritance, their individual behaviours and their relationships to other people, society and the environment. Although access to healthcare is a visible and highly emotional focus in discussions around the determinants of people's health, this book is concerned with those factors – the majority – that create the conditions for health and wellbeing, and are laid down long before anyone sees a healthcare professional. These relate to, for example: the quality of homes families have access to and can afford to live in; the types of green and public spaces that people have access to and can use to exercise and move around safely; the air students breathe around their schools; or the type of food shops children and adults are exposed to as they go to school and work. These are key environmental determinants.

Spatial planning puts these determinants in context. These determinants will vary between places, communities and individuals, as each place, each community, each individual and each group of individuals will have different needs. Public health professionals can help identify these needs, while the spatial planning system can help accommodate them or, at least, to coordinate development across the built and natural environment sectors. Promoting equity in the process is essential, as no one individual or community will be affected by the health determinants in equal measure. That is why it is so important for the concept of health inequalities to be central to the practice of public health spatial planning.

This part of the book provides this context setting and core knowledge for everyone involved in shaping places and communities. It reflects on and refreshes understanding of the determinants of what influences people's physical and mental health and wellbeing, based on recent research, the professions and disciplines involved in addressing these determinants, and the progress that has been made, which is key to improving the practice of spatial planning for health. Professionals from spatial planning and public health sectors have integral and meaningful roles to play, and arguably have a responsibility to work together to deliver healthy places for communities. This part enables readers to:

- understand and be signposted to the existing evidence and literature base for relevant determinants of health for planning (see Chapter 1);
- identify the professional and institutional contexts in which public health spatial planning takes place (see Chapter 2); and
- understand the state of the union between spatial planning and public health, as well as the key themes arising from current practice (see Chapter 3).

Part I key takeaways

- The environment is made up of a diverse range of social, economic and environmental factors that impact on the health and wellbeing of individuals and communities, with more deprived neighbourhoods experiencing less favourable conditions.
- There is a robust public health evidence base to guide planners on those elements of neighbourhood and community design that support

improved health outcomes, and to build in health throughout the planning process.

- Strategies to tackle public health challenges will only be fully realised if the planning and design of the environment are addressed as part of the wider system of legal frameworks and policy directives at the strategic and local levels.
- There is an opportunity to ensure public health professionals and planners have the right competencies to know what they can do about improving health through their respective responsibilities.

1

Evidence case for action

The built environment affects us all. The planning,
design, management and maintenance of the built
environment has a long-term impact upon people
and communities. It is widely acknowledged that
the quality of life, prosperity, health and wellbeing
of an individual is heavily influenced by the 'place'
in which they live or work.

House of Lords (2016, p 3)

Of the many socio-demographic changes that have taken place
over the past 150 years, three stand out as crucial for this book: the
significant increase in the world's population to some 7.8 billion
people today; the movements of people from rural communities
into urban areas, such that more than half of the world's population
now live in cities and urban communities; and the rapid
improvements in health, as observed in increased life expectancy.
Although these changes have taken place at a different pace and
time across the world, almost all countries have experienced
these changes. They have had significant impacts on both rural
communities and urban areas alike, and it is worth reflecting on
how the built and natural environment of neighbourhoods, towns
and cities impacts on health and wellbeing.

Wider determinants of health

The World Health Organization (WHO) recognises that
a diverse range of non-medical factors impact directly and

indirectly on people's health and wellbeing. These are called the 'wider determinants of health' and are the conditions in which people are born, grow, work, live and age. They are part of the wider set of forces and systems shaping the conditions of daily life, and recognise that the 'causes' of good or poor health are the result of a complex interplay of biological, behavioural, social, economic, commercial and environmental factors.

These wider factors impact on individuals in different ways, depending on, for example, their age and genetic inheritance. In turn, such biological factors are mediated by people's behaviours and lifestyle choices, as well as by other socio-economic factors, such as education levels, employment, job security, types of work, income and social networks. Other factors in the environment, such as housing conditions, transportation networks and sanitation systems, also directly or indirectly impact on health to influence our behaviours and our abilities to choose or maintain healthy lifestyles to a greater or lesser extent.

Health and wellbeing are thus impacted by factors outside of healthcare systems and influenced by such factors as spatial planning, the economy and governmental decisions, plans and policies (Marmot et al, 2010; Geddes et al, 2011). These wider determinants of health are multifaceted and need to be addressed in order to tackle the 'causes of the causes' of ill health (Braveman and Gottlieb, 2014; Health Foundation, 2018), which are often policy driven.

The wider determinants of health were conceptualised by Dahlgren and Whitehead (2007). Barton and Grant (2006) developed that framework to illustrate more clearly the impact that the built and natural environment, or 'place', have on health and wellbeing (see Figure 1.1).

Figure 1.1 illustrates how such factors as lifestyle, behaviours and social networks (lighter rings) impact on people based on their age and genetic inheritance (at the centre). These activities are themselves shaped by the local built and natural environment in the place where people live (darker rings), as well as the wider macroeconomic and political climate. The framework also recognises that in a world of climate change, wider planetary forces affecting local environmental conditions are at work that increasingly impact on people's health.

Figure 1.1: The determinants of health and wellbeing in our neighbourhoods

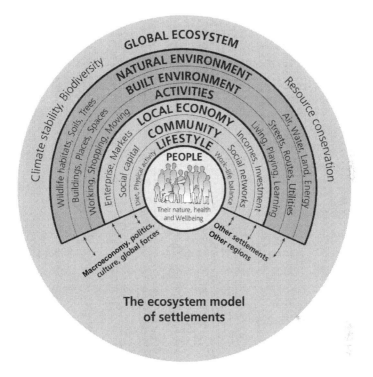

Source: Barton and Grant (2006), developed from a concept by Dahlgren and Whitehead

In other words, your health is largely determined by:

- who you are (person: your age and genetic heredity);
- what you do (behaviour: your individual lifestyle and behaviours [Do you smoke, stay active, or have a job, education and social networks?]); and
- where you live (place: whether the local environment supports healthy living).

The focus of this book is on *'where you live'* and how those factors in the built and natural environment, such as housing conditions, transportation networks and access to green spaces, impact on health directly or indirectly by influencing behaviours and people's abilities to choose and maintain healthy lifestyles.

An emerging body of evidence has been produced showing how the built and natural environment impacts on everyone's health and wellbeing (Townshend, 2022). It can support the establishment of social networks, the location and quality of housing, and exposure to air and noise pollution. The design of houses, estates and connecting roads can, in turn, promote or preclude good connectivity within a neighbourhood, the creation of a safe and accessible transport system, and the support of active travel.

Definition of active travel

Active travel means 'making journeys by physically active means, like walking or cycling. These are usually short journeys, like walking to the shops, walking the kids to school, cycling to work, or cycling to the station to catch a commuter train ... This in turn increases levels of physical activity' (Cavill et al, 2019, p 5). Physical activity is crucial to maintaining health and wellbeing.

The design of urban spaces also plays a crucial role in promoting access to open space, employment and healthy food options. People living in deprived communities within a few miles of each other can experience over ten-year differences in life expectancy (Marmot et al, 2020a; Turnbull, 2021). If public health policy does not pay sufficient attention to the impacts of the built environment on health and wellbeing, key health goals will not be achieved.

Lung disease: an example of how these pathways can affect health

Inflammation and irritation of the lungs are the biological basis underpinning many severe respiratory illnesses (such as asthma). The causes triggering or exacerbating this biological response may come from living in a cold, damp home or from exposure to a range of other pollutants, both within the home and from the wider environment. These, in turn, may arise from poor design, ageing infrastructure or nearby roads clogged with polluting automotive vehicles. Traffic volumes and concerns about air pollution and safety might, in turn, influence people's decision to take a walk and get exercise, or allow children to cycle to school.

People's ability to take effective action about these stressors, that is, to identify and then remedy the underlying causes, might be influenced by their level of education or level of income, for example, being able to pay to insulate or heat a cold home. Taking action at an individual level by altering behaviour may be impossible to achieve if the source of the pollution arises from situations beyond a person's immediate control, for example, a nearby development emitting polluting particles into the air. There is a complex dynamic involved in how the built environment helps shape health by impacting on the ability to make personal choices.

Healthy places, healthy people: health, wellbeing and the environment

A fundamental premise of this book is that many of the health challenges facing modern societies today are mediated through the quality of the built and natural environment. At its most basic level, access to good sanitation, clean drinking water, decent housing and other infrastructure is taken as a given in modern, industrialised countries. This was recognised and identified some 150 years ago by the first urban planners, engineers, medics and statisticians who would, over time, become public health professionals.

At that time, the main causes of death were communicable diseases, such as tuberculosis, typhoid and typhus, whose ease of transmission related to the lack of sanitation, overcrowding and poor housing, which were further exacerbated by poverty, poor nutrition and lack of education and stable jobs. The work of the early urban planners led to better housing and sanitation. The impact of modern medicine, including vaccinations, and increased national wealth led to many of the communicable disease health scourges being brought under control, resulting in a healthier population, living much longer lives (McKeown and Lowe, 1974).

Notwithstanding the COVID-19 pandemic, in most industrialised countries, the communicable diseases of the past have largely been replaced by chronic, non-communicable diseases (NCDs), such as heart disease, stroke, cancer and diabetes. In Europe, NCDs account for almost 90 per cent of deaths – with many of these classified as 'premature' deaths (occurring among those aged between 30 and 70) (WHO, 2022). Significantly, most of these premature deaths from NCDs are due to *modifiable environmental factors* and can be prevented or delayed (WHO, 2013a; Prüss-Ustün et al, 2016) by many measures that can be taken in both lower-income and wealthier countries to reduce disease through better urban planning and design. In England, the leading behavioural causes of years of life lost from NCDs – tobacco use, unhealthy diet, alcohol consumption and physical inactivity – show a relationship with deprivation (Marteau et al, 2021). In 2007, Rao and colleagues examined how the design, availability and maintenance of the built environment influence a range of physical and social features that, in turn, can affect both physical and mental health and wellbeing (see Figure 1.2).

An extensive array of diseases and medical conditions were identified as having some of their underlying causes related to the built environment. Diseases and conditions including asthma, depression, accidents, cardiovascular disease, obesity, infectious diseases, musculoskeletal problems, some forms of cancer and risk factors underlying other diseases, such as lack of physical activity, were also identified.

Figure 1.3 illustrates how urban and transport policies can impact directly and indirectly on health (Nieuwenhuijsen, 2016). The framework illustrates the pervasive impact that the design of the built environment (for example, transport infrastructure and green spaces) can have on health and wellbeing. The availability and design of urban areas' 'walkability' or 'bikeability' will influence people's behaviour as to whether to walk or cycle (active travel), or travel by public

Figure 1.2: The impacts of the built environment on health

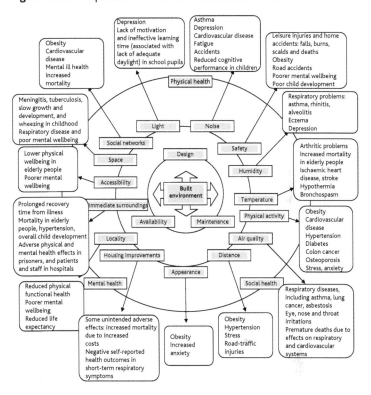

Source: Rao et al (2007)

transport or use cars. These choices, in turn, will have a range of health impacts on both the individual (physical activity) and the community level (contributing to air or noise pollution) (Glazener et al, 2021).

The design of the built and natural environment can help bind neighbourhoods together or sever communities from each other, thereby influencing the establishment of social networks that support reductions in health inequalities (RTPI, 2014; Geddes et al, 2011; Bird et al, 2018). It can support good mental health and wellbeing with green spaces and parks made readily accessible (PHE, 2020c). It also plays a crucial role in promoting access to other features supporting good health, such as education, employment and access to healthy foods,

Figure 1.3: Built environment impacts directly and indirectly on health

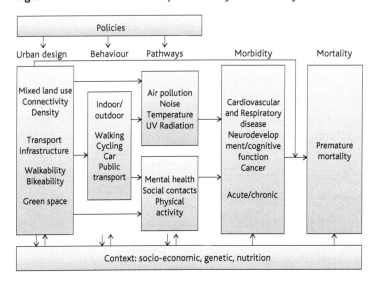

Source: Nieuwenhuijsen (2016)

or preventing health harms, such as exposure to air and noise pollution and road danger.

Poor environment, poor health, more inequality

Although most people are living longer than ever before, differences in life expectancy between different social groups and areas are widening. Almost everywhere, a direct relationship is found between poor environmental conditions and levels of area deprivation, including poor health. Moreover, the distribution of environmental hazards to health is not equal. Those living in the most deprived neighbourhoods are exposed to a greater set of socio-economic and environmental conditions detrimental to health (Marmot et al, 2020a).

Definition of health inequalities

Health inequalities are the unfair and avoidable differences in health status seen within and between countries. All countries demonstrate a social gradient between health and illness: the lower the socio-economic position, the worse the health. Furthermore, poorer health status is generally observed in more deprived localities.

There are significant differences in life expectancy observed between the most deprived and the least deprived localities in even the wealthiest countries. Figure 1.4 shows that in England, a gap of 9.5 years in male life expectancy is observed between those living in the most deprived areas and those living in the least deprived areas. For women, there is nearly an eight-year difference.

Such health inequalities are more pronounced when comparing the number of years of life lived in good health (healthy life expectancy). On average, healthy life expectancy differs by 19 years for both men and women between the most and least deprived local authorities (PHE, 2021). A range of other factors, such as income, education and ethnicity, need to be taken into account when examining the data, but a consistent picture emerges: the places in which people live play a significant role in determining their exposure to health hazards and shaping their behaviours. The result is that 'those in more deprived areas spend a larger proportion of their already shorter lives in poor health' (Marteau et al, 2021, p 1).

Figure 1.4: Differences in life expectancy by area deprivation and sex in England, 2016–18

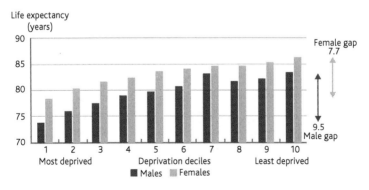

Source: Marmot et al (2020a)

Unhealthy places

Key outcomes observed for people living in the most deprived areas compared to those living in the less deprived areas are as follows:

- *Obesity and nutrition*: associated with an increased risk of a number of common causes of disease and death, including diabetes, cardiovascular disease and some cancers:
  - there are higher densities of fast-food outlets in more deprived areas and a higher prevalence of obesity (Marteau et al, 2021), and obesity is almost twice as likely (NHS Digital, 2018).
- *Physical activity*: contributes to a wide range of health benefits. Regular physical activity can improve health outcomes (irrespective of weight loss):
  - activity levels in adults decrease from 72 per cent active in the least deprived areas to 57 per cent in the most deprived areas (NHS Digital, 2019).
- *Green spaces*: associated with higher self-reported health and mental wellbeing. They can help bring communities together, reduce loneliness and mitigate the negative effects of air pollution, heat and flooding:
  - the most affluent 20 per cent of wards in England have five times the amount of parks or general green space compared with the most deprived 10 per cent of wards (PHE, 2020c).
- *Housing*: a healthy, suitable and stable home environment is essential for people's health and wellbeing throughout their life:
  - 29 per cent of health inequalities can be explained by poor-quality housing and neighbourhood environment (EuroHealthNet, 2019), and in England, 17 per cent or 4.1 million homes failed to meet the Decent Homes Standard (MHCLG, 2020).
- *Road traffic*: road safety prevents injuries and deaths, and has a positive impact on other areas of public health:
  - children in the 10 per cent most deprived wards are four times more likely to be hit by a car than those in the 10 per cent least deprived, and similar inequalities are observed for pedestrian casualties in other age groups too (PHE, 2016).
- *Environmental hazards*: air pollution and noise pollution levels are, on average, worse in areas of highest deprivation:

- in England, 55 per cent of all *carcinogenic chemicals* are released in the 20 per cent most deprived areas (Walker et al, 2003).
- *Crime*: whether or not people feel safe in their neighbourhood and in control in their communities can have physical and psychological effects:
  - victims of crime and offenders are more likely to live in England's most deprived areas than in better-off areas (Marmot et al, 2020a).

Building the evidence base for planning healthy places

A detailed examination of what is scientific evidence and detailed hierarchies of evidence is beyond the scope of this book. From a spatial public health practitioner's perspective, the challenge is to guide planning decisions based on comprehensive and reliable evidence about the effectiveness and costs of alternative strategies (Littell and White, 2018) from robust studies that minimise bias (Campbell Collaboration, 2022).

Figure 1.5 is an example showing the 'hierarchy of evidence' pyramid. This is not a comprehensive list; other types of studies not included here, such as long-term longitudinal monitoring studies or qualitative studies, are also in the researcher's armoury. As one progresses up the pyramid from anecdotal observations or lived experiences to more controlled studies, the emerging evidence generally increases in its reliability or validity of results. For more information about evidence hierarchies, refer to resources published by the Cochrane Collaboration (2022) and the Campbell Collaboration (2022).

Figure 1.5: Hierarchy of evidence used to relate published medical information

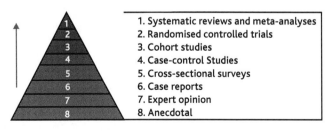

1. Systematic reviews and meta-analyses
2. Randomised controlled trials
3. Cohort studies
4. Case-control Studies
5. Cross-sectional surveys
6. Case reports
7. Expert opinion
8. Anecdotal

Source: Evans and Boyce (2008)

In epidemiology, observational studies that show associations between two factors are crucially important to gain a better understanding of a problem. For example, rates of obesity are twice as prevalent in more deprived areas than less deprived areas, but this observation does not tell us what it is in these areas that is contributing to rates of obesity and what needs to be done to have an impact on such rates. Epidemiologists would then usually subject this to a study controlling for different factors to see what features in the physical environment and other factors are contributing to the observed differences.

In seeking to understand complex problems, such as the impact of the built environment on health, it is not enough to rely on a single observation or controlled study. This will not provide sufficient guidance for policy or practice (Littell and White, 2018). Practitioners have developed a range of techniques and study designs (for example, randomised controlled trials, systematic reviews, meta-analyses and so on) to reduce bias and increase the power or reliability of studies, as well as to ensure transparency and replicability, especially when trying to determine causation (Rosenberg and Donald, 1995; Higgins et al, 2021).

Using an analogy from clinical medicine, in an ideal situation, a medical practitioner will be aware of the best available evidence. In a real-life situation, they will use this information to inform their clinical judgement based on their experience with other patients, taking into account their knowledge of the patient in front of them and the values and preferences of the patient themselves. Overall, this illustrates how evidence-based medicine is practised, as shown in Figure 1.6.

A similar analogy can be drawn for the public health practitioner challenged with developing a public health measure at the population and community levels. It is not just hard scientific 'evidence' on which decisions on treatments or public health policies are based (Woodbury and Kuhnke, 2014), and the literature tends to use the term 'evidence-informed practice or policy'.

For policymakers and planners, and for taking planning decisions more generally, the challenge is perceived somewhat differently. When planners refer to the 'evidence base', they are generally

Figure 1.6: Evidence-based medicine

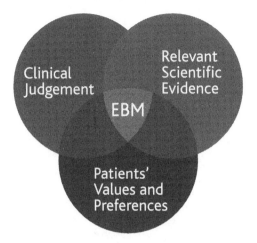

Note: EBM = evidence-based medicine

Source: Morley et al (2019)

referring to information that has been shown to support the objectives of the planning system, as set out in national and local planning policy and regulations, and that has been substantiated by relevant case law and appeal decisions (see Figure 1.7).

In coming to a planning decision, research evidence is only one of many factors – and not necessarily near the top of the pyramid – that will have a significant impact. Public health spatial planners must try to provide the best data and evidence available to support evidence-informed decision-making, as it will be applied in a real 'place'. Their aim is to help decision-makers take planning decisions in the knowledge of the likely impacts that these will have on health and wellbeing.

One of the pioneers of modern public health practice, Archie Cochrane (1972), set out the challenges for evaluating policies and services:

- Is it effective? (Does it work?)
- Is it efficient? (Is it being delivered economically?)
- Is it equitable? (Is it fair?)

Figure 1.7: Policymakers' hierarchy of evidence

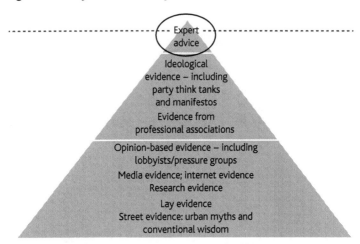

Source: Hunter (2017)

Although the nature of the 'evidence base' may have a somewhat different meaning for the two professions, if the purpose of planning is to contribute to the achievement of sustainable development, with a social objective 'to support strong, vibrant and healthy communities' (MHCLG, 2021b), as in England, then the central questions that Cochrane posed for health services policy can be applied to planning issues.

Using the evidence base for planning healthy places

What is a healthy place?

A healthy place is one that supports and promotes healthy behaviours and environments and a reduction in health inequalities for people of all ages. It will provide the community with opportunities to improve their physical and mental health, and support community engagement and wellbeing. It is a place that is inclusive and promotes social interaction ... It meets the needs of children and young people to grow and develop, as well as being adaptable to the needs of an increasingly elderly population and those with dementia and other sensory or mobility impairments. (MHCLG, 2019)

How might this interpretation of a healthy place translate into practice? For example, exposure to a green space has a range of health benefits:

- promoting healthy behaviours (for example, physical activity and outdoor recreation);
- mediating potential health harms (air pollution, urban heat island and flood mitigation);
- improving social contacts (bringing communities together and creating a sense of inclusion); and
- leading to better academic performance, improved concentration and behaviour. (PHE, 2020c)

It is also observed that many deprived communities have much less access to green spaces. Although this does not necessarily prove causation, improving access to green spaces can support improved health and wellbeing, and give public health teams a base on which to advise spatial planners on how to design for health.

An increasing number and breadth of studies have also provided supporting evidence showing those features of a well-designed environment that will support better health and wellbeing, which can, in turn, be used in planning (Turnbull, 2021). For example, evidence has been provided as to how close to a housing estate urban green space needs to be to ensure that local people will use it often enough to have enough 'exposure' to reap health benefits (Natural England, 2021). Furthermore, as one high-quality review noted: 'Results from this study provide supportive evidence regarding the use of *certain* UGS [urban green space] interventions for health, social and environmental benefits, *in particular* park-based and greenway/trailbased interventions employing a dual approach' (Hunter et al, 2019).

Other recent systematic reviews provide broadly consistent messages on the positive benefits of good design and health, covering a wide range of issues, such as buildings, transport, active travel and health (Stappers et al, 2018; Cavill et al, 2019; Ige et al, 2019), physical activity (Tcymbal et al, 2020), mental health (Núñez-González et al, 2020), green space (Moore et al, 2018; Rojas-Rueda et al, 2019), and health inequalities (McGowan et al, 2021).

Clearly, the built environment can be planned and designed in ways that promote better health and wellbeing for individuals and the communities in which they live. The challenge for public health practitioners and policymakers is to interpret the key messages emerging from the evidence base, while for urban designers and planners, it is to translate these into practical policies, designs and developments in specific places that comply with and balance the views arising from the community, professionals, policies and statutes in the context of political and economic realities (Hunter et al, 2019).

An evidence review identified those design features that are positively associated with better health or had adverse influences on poor health, which were, in turn, published and applied by Public Health England (PHE, 2017) to support spatial planners. In the evidence resource for spatial planning and health, PHE (2017) set out five themes to support a healthy place-making agenda:

1. Neighbourhood design:
   • Complete, compact and walkable neighbourhoods, with good connectivity and safe and efficient infrastructure, can lead to increased physical activity across all ages (the 'life course'), as well as increased social participation among older adults.
   • Developments that prioritise access to such assets as schools, recreational centres and social amenities can increase physical activity across the life course, and the provision of local amenities can improve mobility and social engagement among older adults.
2. Housing:
   • Quality housing can improve health and wellbeing outcomes across the life course, as well as social outcomes among older adults.
   • Provision of affordable housing for those with specific health or social needs can lead to improved quality of life, physical health and mental wellbeing.

3. Food environment:
   - Increased access to healthy, affordable food is associated with improved attitudes towards healthy eating, healthier food-purchasing behaviour and the maintenance of a healthy weight.
4. Natural environment:
   - Improving the quality of parks can increase visitation, usage and physical activity among children and older adults, and access to and engagement with the natural environment is associated with numerous positive health and wellbeing outcomes.
   - Clean air can lead to positive changes in people's health behaviours, with improved air quality associated with increased physical activity among older adults.
5. Transport:
   - Infrastructure to support walking, cycling, active travel and the use of public transport, including road-safety measures, can increase physical activity levels across people's life course.

Concluding statement

It has long been recognised that living in poor environments can have significant health consequences, for example, poor sanitation, poor air quality and cold, damp housing. Research has now begun to show other ways in which the built environment impacts on health and wellbeing, both directly and indirectly. The planning and design of the public realm will support or hinder the ability of people to adopt healthier lifestyles, or will significantly influence their exposure to hazards in the environment. Furthermore, evidence shows that the distribution of risks to health across localities arising from poor environmental conditions, such as lack of access to green spaces or below standard housing, is not equal and is a factor leading to the significant disparities and inequalities in health outcomes observed between deprived and less deprived communities.

Public health has begun to collect an increasingly rich and robust array of evidence to be able to identify with greater confidence those aspects of the built environment and its design that can support people to lead healthier lives. This evidence base can be used to underpin planning decisions in the knowledge that certain actions, designs and developments will help promote better health in the community.

Built environment professionals in both the public and commercial sector and local communities themselves now have the evidence to make the case for urban planning decisions that are good for health. The climate crisis makes these issues all the more urgent to address now.

The challenge is now to ensure that health improvement becomes a fundamental design principle underpinning all planning decisions and that spatial planning, housing, transport, leisure, environment and health teams are mobilised locally to address the wider determinants of health. Unless this is done, wider health issues and health inequalities stand no chance of being successfully tackled.

2

Policy and professional skills context

Spatial planning policy, public health policy and professional priorities have reached a point of convergence that supports the growing movement to reunite planning and health. There remains an inherent complexity in the way those working across the different professions, sectors and parts of civil society interact to shape the places in which we live, work and play, whether in urban or rural communities. Practitioners are experimenting with creative ways to work within local circumstances and systems to deliver on the priorities that matter most to local communities. So there is a need to capture and create an institutional memory of the journey to improve the actions taken to improve health through planning.

This chapter captures the knowledge of practitioners working within current legislative, policy and professional competency frameworks to tackle the challenging public health issues facing this and future generations. It will highlight:

• what is meant by spatial planning and the public health spatial planning paradigms; and
• reframing the public benefit roles of the professional – the planning, public health and wider built environment workforce groups.

Evolution of spatial planning for health

The origins of spatial planning for health began with an understanding of the opportunities that the system and process of spatial planning bring to improve people's health and wellbeing through addressing their environmental determinants. Although there is not a straightforward sequence, our proposition is that there are three phases in spatial planning for health practice that can operate at any one point in time, setting or policy context:

- first phase: health protection;
- second phase: health promotion and improvement; and
- third phase: health inequality reduction.

During the *first phase*, poor environmental conditions in towns and cities resulted in the prevalence of communicable diseases, such as tuberculosis and cholera, and their transmission through the population. Prominent figures include John Snow, who established the link between poor water quality and cholera outbreaks in the late 19th century through detailed mapping studies, though the underlying biological mechanisms for this link were not established until many years later. This prompted action to sanitise neighbourhoods and provide healthier housing and living conditions in order to protect people from such diseases through a combination of novel legislation (such as the Housing and Town Planning Act 1909) and improved urban sanitation works.

A prominent planning approach during this time was Ebenezer Howard's Garden Cities, which were planned to maximise healthy living, and was a concept transposed across the globe, for example, in the Netherlands, the US and Japan (Geertse, 2008). A pamphlet written by Dr Norman Macfadyen, the chair of the Garden Cities and Town Planning Association, as well as Letchworth Garden City's first chief medical officer in 1938, summarised the essence of healthy living as attributable to 'good housing conditions, good working conditions, good opportunity for the enjoyment of leisure, freedom for proper rest, with the proper opportunity for fresh food' (Macfadyen, 2013, p 7). These are (some of) the wider determinants of health as we define them today.

While modern society takes for granted advancements in infectious disease control, many of the practices to prevent and manage infections and contaminations continue today through the work of environmental health officers, healthcare practitioners, architects and designers in certain settings, for example, in food-preparation premises and in health and care buildings (Department of Health, 2013).

The legislative origins of planning for health in the UK since 1947

In the UK post-war period, the introduction of a formal system for managing the built environment for the health and betterment of the population saw the establishment of the planning system with the Town and Country Planning Act 1947 (TCPA, 2017), together with the establishment of the National Health Service (NHS) with the NHS Act 1946.

During the *second phase* in the late 20th and early 21st centuries, there was a more sophisticated understanding of the determinants of health and the role of planning, including a greater focus on specific sectors and the issues and needs of population groups, such as ageing, children and young people, and promoting physical activity. Institutions and practitioners began to grapple with the further assimilation of specific public health issues by gaining a better technical understanding and working knowledge of the planning powers and levers available to relevant municipal institutions. Part II provides an example of the interdisciplinary use of HIAs and environmental assessments for plans and projects.

Healthy urban planning in the WHO European Healthy Cities Network

The WHO European Healthy Cities network offers an insight into the evolutionary journey of planning for health through its various programme phases. For example, themes in Phase IV (2003–08) and Phase V (2009–13) focused on planning/health processes, such as healthy urban design and planning, while the later Phase VI (2014–18) focused on specific health issues, such as ageing, physical activity, obesity and mental health.

An example is the Belfast Healthy Cities designation in Phase V of the WHO European Healthy Cities Network (2009–13), which included a workstream on healthy urban environments. An online resource on reuniting planning and health was also developed with the TCPA to inform and support specific areas for action. It includes examples of good practice from Northern Ireland, the UK and elsewhere in Europe (Belfast Healthy Cities, 2014).

As we move further through the 21st century during the *third phase*, in addition to the accumulation of knowledge and experience from previous phases, health inequalities and equity become the dominant theme and focus of all practitioners. In some national legislative frameworks, there are increasingly explicit references to reducing health inequalities as a legal responsibility in the functions of institutions and agencies, such as PHE in the UK and, more locally, the Liverpool City Region Combined Authority. Many professional bodies' codes of conduct for their members now require competencies on ethics and equality.

This 'evolutionary' process has meant that these phases are concurrently in play as professionals and institutions adapt and interchange in response to local circumstances, such as those now facing wealthier and poorer nations. Spatial planning for health has established itself as a paradigm that can:

- inspire a health vision for the future of places that responds to both local challenges of inequalities and local opportunities;
- translate this vision into a set of priorities, programmes, policies and land-use decisions, with the resources and resolve to deliver on them;
- create a framework for public–private investment that promotes economic, environmental and social health and wellbeing;
- coordinate the actions and priorities of key agencies and processes; and
- contribute to the achievement of the UN SDGs, including on good health and wellbeing (SDG3) and reduced inequalities (SDG10).

Spatial planning

'Spatial planning' is a catch-all term that refers to all levels of a system that manages land-use activities to meet the needs of society, the economy and the environment. These levels can include national government departments responsible for setting policy or direct infrastructure development, and local government institutions responsible for guiding decisions on urban development schemes promoted by private sector interests or for which they are directly responsible. Spatial planning can also be referred to as a process that sets out what these key socio-economic and environmental ingredients are, how and when they should be translated into actions, and by whom.

Permutations of the term 'spatial planning'

Spatial planning can also be known as: 'planning', 'land-use planning', 'urban planning', 'town planning', 'city planning', 'town and country planning' and 'territorial planning'. How the term is used can vary from country to country. Practitioners should not be confused by the variety of ways in which the term is used internationally and interchangeably. Aside from nuances indicated in respective legislative and policy frameworks, there are no fundamental differences regarding its application in practice.

The system and process of spatial planning can best be understood as comprising four components within a framework, as set out in Table 2.1. Within each of these, it is important that health and wellbeing issues are embedded throughout to ensure that town and urban developments are guided by such considerations.

Legal framework

Many countries have set out parameters of spatial planning practice in legislation. The importance of legal underpinning for spatial planning activities should not be understated, as it sets out the purpose, objective, functions, stakeholders, outcomes of

Table 2.1: Planning components and scope of health considerations

Component	Spatial scale	Scope of health consideration
Legal framework	International or national	• Set mandatory objectives for bodies and their functions in protecting and improving health. • Enable permissive powers and procedures for considering health.
Strategic policy directive	National or regional	• Set an express policy basis and encourage necessary levers for achieving health.
Local policy directive	Local or neighbourhood	• Detail localised policy basis and guide the necessary levers for achieving health.
Development management	Site or building	• Manage the application of policy and levers for achieving health.

functions and enforcement through legal processes. Town and country planners must work within the law or can suffer the consequences of not doing so, with decisions being challenged through local judicial or quasi-judicial processes. This is why planners often cite statutory provisions or case law, in addition to relying on academic literature, in practice.

The legal framework also provides the necessary powers and levers, and frames the scope and limits of their application in practice. Examples include but are not limited to: achieving certain public interest objectives, such as reducing health inequalities; working towards sustainable development; undertaking HIAs; statutory duties to achieve specified outcomes; and processes of statutory consultation and engagement with stakeholders. When these are introduced and defined in legal frameworks, they are afforded a much higher and stronger degree of imposition and compliance (Nau et al, 2021).

This quasi-legal basis of planning activity is adapted to the way public health and the medical profession operate. However, the opportunity exists to ensure legal frameworks enable and support, not hinder or discount, the practice of planning for health, and that planners have a competent understanding and knowledge of where such opportunity exists to help achieve public health objectives.

Strategic policy directive

Governmental departments and agencies will set out policies as national directives to enact the legal parameters of legislation. It is often in this component where the aspirations and expectations of governments in relation to planning are clearly expressed. These can be in the form of a statement, strategy or action plan, policy requirements or standards, and technical guidance. This is usually at the highest tier of the decision-making hierarchy. Depending on the institutional governance arrangements of countries, this may be at national, state, regional or provincial levels.

They form the basis of the further policy development and decision-making of lower-tier local institutions and agencies, and often require a degree of conformity and accountability. It should be noted that policies at this level have to be applicable across a wide range of scenarios and therefore project a sense of strategic clarity and consistency.

Strategic policy directives can also provide the necessary policy powers and levers, and frame the scope and limits of their application. Examples include the use of travel plans, undertaking certain assessments and development standards or benchmarks. When these are introduced and defined in policy directives, they are afforded a proportionate degree of compliance, though less so than if they were set out in legal frameworks.

In practice, different powers and levers are introduced in either legal or policy frameworks, depending on the degree of political commitment to the issues. Legal processes require following established parliamentary protocols and often take longer than processes for publishing policies or strategies. There will always be an element of pragmatism in planning practice.

Local policy directive

Municipal institutions at lower-tier levels (sub-regional, municipal or even neighbourhood) have a different jurisdiction and political accountability to those bodies who set strategic policy directives. They may be legally required or empowered to set locally specific policies according to local contexts, circumstances, priorities and needs. While these may often be required to conform and not contravene strategic policy directives, they do provide a level of geographical specificity and location contextualisation necessary to realise the spatial vision of health and wellbeing. This specificity will be justified by a combination of commissioned studies and evidence gathering in both qualitative and quantitative methods, as well as cross-referencing to other non-planning settings, such as public health and healthcare planning.

Development management

Development management in spatial planning refers to the process of administration, that is, determining and managing a development application by the public authority in accordance with legislative and policy requirements. Development management can be considered as the coal face of implementing and applying public health spatial planning practice, where discussions become highly technical and practical, and expectations and aspirations come face to face with political, economic, cultural and professional realities. Strategic and local policy directives set the rules and requirements within which site- or building-specific activities can and should take place in the act of applying for development consent.

The development management process requires planners working in national and local government institutions, along with elected representatives, to apply policies to land-use approvals. Such activities are manifested in a range of projects of varying types of uses and scales (for illustrated examples of these, see Figure 2.1), such as:

• an extension or the building of a single residential building in the rural countryside;
• a residential-led scheme of several hundred units in the form of detached homes and apartment blocks on a metropolitan site of regeneration;
• a commercial scheme of hectares of floorspace of office or warehousing activities; and
• a utilities infrastructure scheme, such as a major road, waste plant, renewable or low-carbon energy project, or airport.

Figure 2.1: Typology of developments where health considerations need to be tailored to

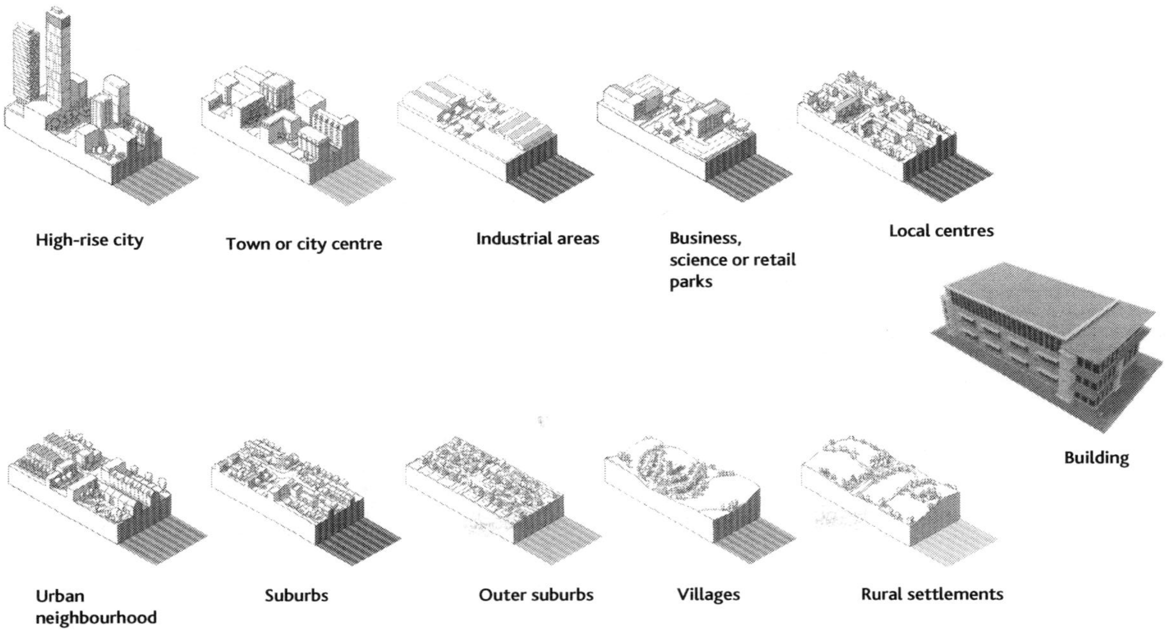

High-rise city

Town or city centre

Industrial areas

Business, science or retail parks

Local centres

Building

Urban neighbourhood

Suburbs

Outer suburbs

Villages

Rural settlements

Source: MHCLG (2021d)

Subsequent chapters will highlight further examples of good practice where, through engagement with relevant stakeholders, practitioners have embedded public health issues into the planning process.

Planning for health professional context

There is increasing recognition that planning, public health and wider built environment professionals are at the forefront of planning for health. Many of their representative professional bodies – in planning, public health, landscape architecture, building and engineering, transportation, and housing – are beginning to update their corporate charters, membership criteria and professional development requirements to consider public interest topics. Most will have competency frameworks against which members must demonstrate their qualifications and experience, and that these are refreshed regularly as part of continuing professional development (CPD). However, the inclusion of public health and wellbeing, inequalities, and equity as core knowledge components generally remains at the discretion of individuals based on their own professional interest, rather than a formal registration requirement.

The UK Built Environment Advisory Group (2018) (a collaboration between four of the UK's built environment professional institutes: the Royal Institute of British Architects, the Royal Town Planning Institute [RTPI], the Institution of Structural Engineers and the Landscape Institute) acknowledged the need for integrated approaches to achieve sustainable outcomes. Their competency frameworks are evolving to include health as part of CPD requirements. However, for now, the public health competency frameworks are more limited, and although the curriculum certainly focuses on the wider determinants of health, it does not contain a specific component on spatial planning and the planning system.

This section identifies the skills, knowledge and behaviours that should be required for the practice of planning for health, whether in public service, private sector commissions or voluntary and community sector advocacy. These skills, knowledge and behaviours seek to supplement and bring together existing education and professional development training curricula, and can be adapted or evolve as new trends, legal requirements, practices and knowledge arise. They fall into three categories:

- technical: providing expertise on specific topics;
- context: setting the expertise in context; and
- delivery and implementation: achieving outcomes as a result.

Who are the practitioners working at this interface and now acquiring and gaining expert status in these competencies? There is more on this in Chapter 9, which introduces the rise of the 'public health spatial planning' practitioner, such as in local government and other public sector authorities. Postgraduate, early-career education and professional development will play an increasingly important role and is also dealt with in Chapter 9 of the book.

Technical

Technical competencies require a degree of ability and expert knowledge of topic areas considered core to the profession and communicating across professions. Demonstrating technical competency is an essential aspect for all professional training, as it provides practitioners with an element of authority and credibility for their actions. This normally includes: knowledge of law and policy requirements, parameters, systems and processes, and ethical considerations; topic-based knowledge, including on sustainable development, public health, obesity, mental health and community development; and skills relating to evidence gathering, analysis and policy development (see Table 2.2). Such action terms as 'develop', 'appraise', 'identify', 'apply', 'critique', 'advise', 'map' and 'collate' are commonly used when describing the competencies.

Context

Context competencies relate to the ability to work with and through the different policy, political, institutional and organisational contexts and settings. They enable circumstantial

Table 2.2: 'Technical' competencies for public health spatial planning in practice

Competency	Skills, knowledge and behaviours
Data and analysis	Systematic collation and analysis of place, population and public health data – needs, risks and trends.
Evidenced decision-making	Information-gathering strategies and thinking processes in making healthy and fair planning decisions.
Impact assessment	Appraisal of health impact of policies and projects, with engagement with experts, researchers and local communities.
Law and policy development	Understanding of the relevant planning and health legal frameworks that underpin practice and compliance.
Urban design and planning	Having spatial and urban design awareness and techniques to visualise and present information, and then recommend planning/design solutions.

actions and decisions to be undertaken, and include efforts to be adaptable and build partnerships, alliances and mutually beneficial collaborations across and within sectors. In many ways, context competencies are grounded in practice and ethical practices. Such action terms as 'facilitate', 'promote', 'influence', 'build', 'translate' and 'connect' are commonly used when describing these competencies (see Table 2.3).

Delivery and implementation

Delivery and implementation competencies enable the necessary action to be undertaken, whether it relates to policy development, programme management or decision taking. Such competencies are critical in making things happen and seeing results on the ground, or at least setting out an approach to plan and manage. Such action terms as 'coordinate', 'initiate', 'deliver', 'influence', 'adapt' and 'track' are commonly used when describing the competencies (see Table 2.4).

Although having such a range of competencies is ideal and necessary in a competent professional practice in public health

Table 2.3: 'Context' competencies for public health spatial planning in practice

Competency	Skills, knowledge and behaviours
Contemporary practice	Understanding of planning and health, and their integrated healthy cities and environments systems and frameworks.
Politics in practice	Understanding of the influences of different governance levels of political and democratic processes.
Health leadership advocacy	Promotion of policies and projects through health and wellbeing, health inequalities, and a wider determinants lens.
Cultural change	Facilitation of cultural, institutional or individual professional behavioural changes to planning for health.
Ethics and public interest	Ethical practices when promoting population health and reducing health inequalities.

Table 2.4: 'Delivery and implementation' competencies for public health spatial planning in practice

Competency	Skills, knowledge and behaviours
Multidisciplinary working	Acting with integrity, objectivity and openness in working across and with multiple disciplines, sectors and agencies.
Population engagement	Engaging and involving specific groups and stakeholders in policy, as well as those likely to be affected by interventions.
Communication	Adapting communication techniques for transferring information to different audience, purposes and specific groups.
Development economics	Understanding of real estate development, commercial factors and viability associated with planning interventions.
Programme initiation	Designing place-based programmes and implementing solutions to support population level health and wellbeing.
Evaluation and review	Application of techniques and strategies for the monitoring of policies and projects, and recommendations for review.

spatial planning, challenges remain, in particular, in upskilling the existing workforce. As competency frameworks are refreshed and updated to reflect changing priorities and opportunities, they primarily benefit new and recently trained and accredited professionals. Established and long-standing members may have been trained and accredited in different technical and contextual competencies.

Learning and professional development

Learning and development are dynamic, not a static state. In practice, a combination of these competencies is required, and professionals will call upon them as and when necessary to achieve outcomes. Certainly, each of the competency categories in themselves will not be sufficient to demonstrate competency, as was eloquently articulated when Macfadyen (2013, p 5) reflected on contemporary limitations on planning for health, stating: 'The specialist knows "more and more about less and less" and we get quite lost, and acquire a materialistic outlook on things.' An overreliance on technical specialists will not address many of the complex issues society faces, where the softer context competencies can be more effective.

Gaining and applying these skills requires all professionals to continually improve through reflective practice and the self-management of learning and development; therefore, professional bodies often require all members to undertake, record and reflect on their CPD activities each year. These institutions allow their members to self-determine what CPD is relevant to their practice and learning needs, and the format and method, as long as they also meet competency frameworks.

CPD requirements

In the planning profession, chartered or certified planners in the UK with the RTPI are required to undertake a minimum of 50 hours over a two-year period, while certified US planners with the American Institute of Certified Planners (AICP) are required to undertake 32 credits or 32 hours over a two-year period. In public health, the UK Faculty of Public Health required its qualified members to complete 50 credits per year, before these requirements were replaced from 1 April 2022 with completion of reflective notes linked to members' professional development plan.

In practice, combining these sets of skills and knowledge, and keeping them up to date through CPD, can help cultivate meaningful working relationships. Productive and transparent relationships where professionals appreciate and respect each other's contributions, and are open to testing and trialling solutions to overcome challenges and barriers, are important.

Concluding statement

The legislative and policy dimension is critical for ensuring that public health spatial planning actions and aspirations are legally compliant and in conformity with the respective jurisdictions of each nation. They may differ from country to country, state to state or authority to authority, depending on the nature of the devolution of powers. Whatever regulatory framework is in place, actions on the built environment and health must be aligned with the wider policy and political commitment to healthy places nationally and regionally, and reflect the priorities of communities. In this way, we will begin to see sustained change in the design of our urban spaces towards ones that are truly health promoting. Seeking a greater union between professionals is critical for professional bodies representing planners and public health practitioners to address and to establish the type of common 'technical', 'context' and 'delivery and implementation' competencies necessary to improve the practice of planning for health.

3

Current state of planning for health

> It will be important to take advantage of existing and new networks to provide multidisciplinary action, both for the planning and design of the built environment and in support of more healthy, equitable, and thriving communities.
>
> McKinnon et al (2020)

This chapter reviews the state of the union and joint working between spatial planning and public health, and the extent to which wider political and research landscapes have influenced this union. As set out in Chapter 1, we know in principle and from evidence 'what works'. What is unknown is how these can be applied in different localities under different conditions through the planning system. The unique, place-based composition of the built and natural environment makes it difficult to develop evidence-based approaches that can be universally applied, and successful practices in one setting may not always be transferrable to another.

This chapter synthesises research from academic and practice-based literature to establish an 'institutional' memory of the planning for health journey. It also illustrates:

- research reviewing the state of the union between spatial planning and public health in practice; and
- those themes that have emerged setting out the range of challenges and opportunities faced by practitioners.

Scope of research into the state of the union

Over the past decade, there has been an emerging body of research and reports reflecting on the state of the union between spatial planning and public health in practice. These have either focused on the strategic union or on specific planning issues, such as obesity, older people, active travel and climate change, mainly conducted by academic research institutes, special interest and professional groups, and parliamentary oversight committees.

Academia

Academic institutions play a critical role in collecting data and information to help evaluate the effect of policies, interventions and practices. They are able to provide the necessary critical thinking, capacity, research methods and independence to provide high-quality and robust, and therefore useful, findings. In particular, as such findings are published in peer-reviewed journals, they are provided with the authority and objectiveness needed to ground and help inform policy and practice. They are also often anchored in localities, either at the regional or local levels, and therefore have established working relationships with agencies, authorities and stakeholders, including those working in public health spatial planning.

Academics have increasingly focused on the effectiveness of the practice of planning for health, and on planning's contribution to addressing major public issues, such as obesity. While this work does not discount the need for continuing research into the evidence base and the effectiveness of environmental interventions in addressing the wider determinants of health, it does increasingly reflect sentiment by practitioners of the need to take action and evaluate the results of such actions.

In order to do better translational research, academics are undertaking mixed-methods activities to identify and better understand the challenges of applying evidence-based planning for health principles into practice at a local policy and project level (for example, at Fuse, the Centre for Translational Research in Public Health). These activities focus on interacting directly with front-line practitioners in local government or the private sector through

Delphi processes, semi-structured interviews, focus groups and targeted surveys. These practitioners work within spatial planning and wider place-based functions, including planning, transport, housing, parks and recreation, environmental health, and public health, and have responsibilities for turning knowledge into action.

WHO Collaborating Centre for Healthy Urban Environments at the University of the West of England

The University of the West of England hosts one of only two WHO collaborating centres in the world situated in a built environment faculty. The Collaborating Centre for Healthy Urban Environments is working to promote the scientific underpinning of the built environment as a determinant of health, wellbeing and equity, and to support capacity-building activities in the WHO's Healthy Cities programme (www.uwe.ac.uk/research/centres-and-groups/who).

Special interest and professional groups

Many key stakeholder groups within the voluntary, community and social enterprise (VCSE) sectors have helped champion and drive the planning for health agenda, even as priorities at the governmental level move and sway with the political tides. Given their direct connection to community interests, voluntary sector organisations play a critical role in acting as thought leaders and helping to raise awareness of significant issues that may not be a high priority or where limited actions are being undertaken. They have expertise and experience in implementing effective and impactful communication and translational research activities to directly reach planning for health professionals, as they often represent or employ such professions and therefore have a good understanding of the right language and outreach methods to use. However, they are often small organisations with limited resources and dependent on the availability of and access to grant funding from governmental or private sector sources.

They have long recognised the 'implementation gap' and the need for action and support for the translation of academic research into deliverable projects on the ground. They also help communicate findings upstream to governments in order to help positively influence non-partisan legislative and policy development, including submitting evidence to parliamentary oversight committee inquiries and governmental consultations on policy announcements.

Parliamentary oversight committees and commissions

Parliamentary and government-initiated commissions play an important role in holding governments to account and can be influential in recommending policy changes and improvements. They are particularly important when actions and investment in healthy places and environment by public sector bodies, local government and the private sector depend on the existence and strength of commitment from the highest level of government or a policymaking body. Most notably, the Royal Commission on Environmental Pollution (RCEP) – set up under royal warrant in 1970 to advise the Queen, governments, Parliament and the public on environmental issues but closed in 2011 – was one of the first organisations to recognise the practice of planning for health in its 2007 report on the urban environment (RCEP, 2007). In it, the RCEP identified good practice approaches to integrating planning and health across the UK and Europe, and indicated that the planning system offers an important opportunity for a more coherent effort to affect positively the health and wellbeing of communities.

UK House of Lords Select Committee on National Policy for the Built Environment

The House of Lords Select Committee on National Policy for the Built Environment was appointed in 2015 to consider the development and implementation of national policy for the built environment, and to make recommendations. Over the course of the inquiry, it received 187 submissions of written evidence, took oral evidence from 58 witnesses and carried out two site visits. Its final report (House of Lords, 2016) made recommendations supporting augmented actions on health and the built environment. In its response to the report, particularly in relation to public health, the UK government noted that, in working with the Department of Health, government departments will determine where planning could be strengthened to assist local areas in their efforts to better integrate health and planning (DCLG, 2016).

The previous sections only provide a snapshot of those with research interests in this dynamic agenda, which is gaining significant political, research and practitioner interest, partly driven by the acute impact of a global pandemic.

Themes on planning for health in practice research

From the body of research activities undertaken and published, there are key themes to convey to readers to improve public health spatial planning practice. While much of the research originates from the UK, their themes are transferable and applicable across different jurisdictions, contexts, countries and cultures.

Ten themes for improving public health spatial planning practice

- Having a strong legislative and policy basis.
- Making the most of the powers and levers available.
- Formalising clear expectations.
- Developing a shared evidence base.
- Considering public health as an explicit factor in planning decision-making.
- Monitoring and evaluating the impact and effect of actions.
- Having political leadership at national and local levels.
- Improving communication among practitioners and to decision-makers.
- Improving professional and institutional capacity building and training.
- Acknowledging the complexity and holistic nature of the agenda.

Having a strong legislative and policy basis

As spatial planning is a quasi-legal process, stakeholders look to legislation and policy directives as reference points. That is why many planning documents begin with statements referencing legislative provisions. There is a clear hierarchy of weight placed on wording that is in legislation versus wording placed in policy directives. While the distinction appears to be minor, the significance in practice should not be underestimated. As a general rule of thumb, where legislation or policy uses the word 'may' or 'can', it confers a power, while the word 'shall' or 'must' imposes a statutory duty and responsibility. If supporting public health objectives or meeting people's health and wellbeing needs are considered part of the core purpose and objective of planning by politicians and practitioners alike, it is important and necessary to articulate this clearly and unambiguously in legislation and policy instruments.

New Zealand legislative framework for planning

The New Zealand Resource Management Act 1991 defines the statutory purpose of planning functions with explicit reference to health and wellbeing in a way that many other countries do not. Planning is about 'managing the use, development, and protection of natural and physical resources in a way, or at a rate, which enables people and communities to provide for their social, economic, and cultural well-being and for their health and safety' (Section 5).

Making the most of the powers and levers available

The planning system presents practitioners with a range of powers and levers that can be creatively adapted to deliver on a range of policy priorities, including obesity and healthy weight (Chang and Radley, 2020). Many powers and levers may be process-oriented requirements, such as the need to conduct a health impact and environmental assessment, while many are based on good practice and discretionary activities, such as design reviews.

There are limitations, as many of these powers and levers will not have been initially designed to apply specifically to tackling public health issues, such as obesity, and practitioners may not have full control of the drivers of such issues. However, the key message is that the practitioners have a range of levers and opportunities to influence them, and can select the most appropriate ones according to the context, purpose and stage in the planning process. Knowledge of planning for health may not necessarily be about knowledge of evidence and data, but be about what powers and levers are available, and testing their limits. Many public authorities have already effectively influenced those functions that impact on health, such as planning, housing and transport (LGA, 2018b).

Planning powers and levers relevant to obesity

In 2018, the UK Department of Health and Social Care commissioned a three-year trailblazer programme to work with English councils to tackle childhood obesity at a local level by taking bold action to harness existing powers and overcome barriers to addressing the childhood obesity challenge (LGA, 2018a). One of the trailblazers, with Blackburn with Darwen Council in Pennine Lancashire, has resulted in working closely with the planning department to use a positive planning approach to granting planning permission to food premises serving healthier food choices and compiling data to create a better understanding of the scale of food premises gaining planning permission in the locality.

Formalising clear expectations

The planning system provides a framework for those involved in developing the public realm through the built environment and usually also provides a framework for how local communities can engage with this process. It is a wide-ranging system, so greater prescription or formalisation at the right levels of legislation and policy would be a helpful and positive enabler. This would also be welcomed by those making investment and capital funding decisions – whether a public body or the private sector – as a measure of certainty, clarity and stability, which can only be beneficial.

Too much prescription can inhibit innovation and timely revision, particularly when new evidence or trends emerge, such as those being experienced as a result of COVID-19 from 2020 onwards. However, expectations can ensure a degree of consistency and regularity to which policies and decisions can look as a reference point, especially as a way to manage the complexity of information and data from research and regulatory guidelines.

Developing a shared evidence base

Setting out clear expectations should be premised on robust and transparent data and intelligence, which can be turned into a shared evidence base for policy development and decision taking. Often, however, the use of public health data as an evidence base in the planning system is highly contested and often disregarded as appropriate evidence. The issues of the local relevance, applicability and consistency of evidence to support policy and decisions will continue to trouble practitioners when seeking to successfully deliver healthier environments through planning (McGill et al, 2015; Ige et al, 2020).

A good starting point is creating a shared evidence base for public health and planning practitioners. Examples of this include the British Columbia Centre for Disease Control's (2018) *Healthy Built Environment Linkages Toolkit*, which describes how population health is influenced by the design of our neighbourhoods, housing, transportation systems, natural environments and food systems, as well as many other municipal governments with frameworks for planning for health. More examples are provided in Chapter 7.

Worcestershire planning for health technical research paper

Public health and planning colleagues in this English county government have worked together on a background technical evidence paper to inform future planning policy and decision-making. Published in 2015, it provides a summary of local health issues and challenges, and identifies the impact of health determinants on the population. The objective is

57

for this work to be used to inform future planning policy and decision-making across the county, including leading to the publication of an HIA toolkit in 2016.

Considering public health as an explicit factor in planning decision-making

In practice, the planning balance during decision-making on urban development schemes or wider debate around the built and natural environments is tilted towards such issues as the costs, quality and wellbeing of a place (Building Better, Building Beautiful Commission, 2019). In order to boost local authorities' effectiveness in planning for health, public health concerns need to take a more central place early in the planning consideration process. This issue has been consistently raised by public health practitioners and parliamentarians, such as in the UK when dealing with obesity (House of Commons Health Select Committee, 2015), who recommend that health issues should be included as an explicit material planning consideration in the planning decision-making process. (Illustrated examples of development cases and further discussion are presented in Chapter 8). Research has shown that the planning system is reinforcing racial inequalities, and while there is equalities legislation in place, considerations are not mainstreamed in practice, particularly in planning to meet the housing needs of minority ethnic groups (Bristow, 2021).

Monitoring and evaluating the impact and effect of actions

'Plan and monitor' is central to both the planning and public health systems but has been and continues to be the weakest link in helping better understand the effect of actions on people's health and wellbeing. This is, in part, because it is challenging to determine cause and effect between a particular planning policy or decision and a health and wellbeing outcome. However, undertaking monitoring and evaluating, or at least setting out a monitoring framework based on a logic model, provides the opportunity to improve future actions.

Healthy New Towns logic models – foundations for evaluation

Each of the 10 demonstrator sites in NHS England's Healthy New Towns programme created a logic model to underpin the relationship between project activities and desired outcomes. The programme guidance, 'Putting health into place' (NHS England, 2019), suggested that although logic models do not capture the complexity of the place, they are a helpful starting point.

Having political leadership

Carmichael et al (2019) explored how practitioners or decision-makers, such as politicians, consider evidence in the decision-making process, including the application of evidence from such policy sources as corporate strategies and national/federal ministerial statements. At the level where planning decisions are usually made in local government, because planning and public health responsibilities are generally assigned to different portfolios and to different committees, planning matters are often absent from public health discourse and vice versa. In this regard, there is also a need to account for political factors and individuals as a contributing and useful driver in planning for health.

Improving communication among practitioners and to decision-makers

The coming together of different professions and disciplines means the need to be aware of and adopt a shared understanding of jargon and working practices. The differences in communication can be seen in the respective strategies and plans produced – planning documents are full of policies, technical supporting text and maps, while public health documents contain data, images and sometimes individual stories about experiences. There is always room for improvement in appropriately communicating planning for health actions, processes and outcomes in different contexts, and planners and public health practitioners must always be mindful of the end user and target audience.

Improving professional and institutional capacity building and training

Resourcing, capacity building and training have been and continue to be consistent themes when seeking to understand the barriers and opportunities of planning for health. Reduced funding across local governments can impact on overall staff numbers, their visibility and accessibility by external and internal stakeholders, and opportunity to invest time and resources in health-promoting initiatives. Identifying those actors and activators working in key sectors in the agenda and bringing them together can cement collaborations and enable more impactful joint actions (for examples, see Figure 3.1).

The TCPA (2019) has identified a rise in specialist posts in the local government workforce, often jointly funded by the public health and the planning, transport or regeneration departments. At the fundamental level and with minimal structural changes needed, there is a need to see how professions can align their competencies to deliver on shared aspirations for healthier environments.

On training, public health and planning professionals undergo structured education and assessment processes to secure academic and professional qualifications. There is an increasing move to deliver shared learning opportunities in order to participate in building knowledge of each other's systems and issues, and the online learning trend accelerated by COVID-19 makes this option even more viable.

Healthy places competency for landscape architects

The UK Landscape Institute's new entry standards and competency framework introduces a new 'core landscape competency on healthy places' (Landscape Institute, 2020). This competency requires a tiered level of capability in adopting 'the principles of healthy places that improve the physical aspects of the landscape (air, water and soil quality)'.

Figure 3.1: Mapping of organisations active in public health spatial planning

Skills and knowledge Professional representative bodies	• American Planning Association • Faculty of Public Health • Institute of Environment Management and Assessment • Landscape Institute • Royal Institute of British Architects • Royal Town Planning Institute
Advocacy and capacity building Special interest groups, networks and non-government organisations	• Center for Active Design • Health and Wellbeing in Planning Network • Housing LIN • International WELL Building Institute • Local Government Association • Place Alliance • Royal Society of Public Health • Town and Country Planning Association • Urban Land Institute • What Works Centre for Wellbeing
Research, evidence and evaluation Academia and research institutions	• Centre for Health Equity Training Research and Evaluation • Environmental Design Research Association • Fuse, Centre for Translational Research in Public Health • Institute of Health Equity, UCL • National Institute for Health and Care Excellence • UK Collaborative Centre for Housing Evidence
Partnership and end user Community, third-sector and social enterprise groups	• Dementia UK • Alzheimer's Society • UK Voluntary Community and Social Enterprise Health and Wellbeing Alliance

On universities and higher education, there is variance between institutions that provide learning and training, ranging from short healthy urban environment modules to formal degree-level qualifications on urban planning and public health. In the former, it is common place for courses in UK universities to offer guest lectures and/or short modules on healthy urban environments, but they may not provide the necessary level of technical competencies to develop and sustain public health spatial planning practice because of the need to understand and be kept up to date on technical policy and legislative requirements. In the latter, such joint degrees are more commonly offered in the US, for example, a joint Master in Urban/City Planning and Master in Public Health (for more details, see Chapter 9).

Acknowledging the complexity and holistic nature of the agenda

Increasingly, research and policy understanding of the issues has pointed to the complexity of implementing planning for health. Promoting a systems approach means no single action or organisation acting alone and having an understanding of the right points where actions can have most impact on health (Black et al, 2021). This makes the task of communicating the issues to policymakers more challenging and implementing actions by practitioners less effective if done without a coherent strategy. There is a need to gain a better understanding of the interconnectedness of the factors that underpin a healthy environment in a more consistent manner in future research programmes and professional practices.

Adopting a whole-systems approach to obesity

A whole-systems approach to obesity is an example of where many actions through the planning system can be possible parts, such as active travel, healthier food environments and green space provision (see Figure 3.2; see also Blackshaw and van Dijk, 2019).

Concluding statement

The integration of planning and health has experienced highs and lows, but there is increasing interest shown across sectors and disciplines in seeing the results of the union come to fruition in terms of improved outcomes for health and wellbeing. While the planning and public health systems undergo reforms, when engagement with stakeholders is at its peak, and when they are more open to discussion and ideas, the opportunity for a 'reset' arises.

Going forward, it is clear that the fundamental understanding and basis already exists but that barriers still exist and the full range of opportunities and possibilities for improvement is up for grabs. Such key terms as 'inequalities', 'Health In All Policies', 'collaboration', 'partnership' and 'whole systems' underpin what

Figure 3.2: Common areas of obesity activity identified as part of a whole-systems approach to obesity

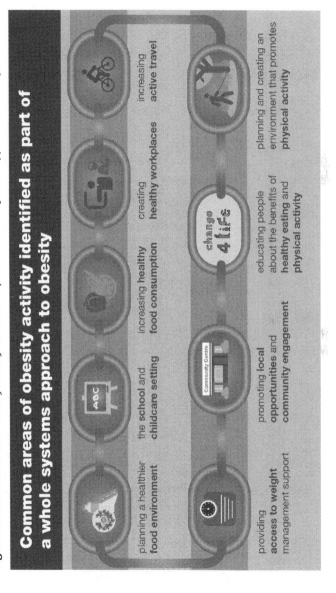

Common areas of obesity activity identified as part of a whole systems approach to obesity

planning a healthier food environment

the school and childcare setting

increasing healthy food consumption

creating healthy workplaces

increasing active travel

planning and creating an environment that promotes physical activity

providing access to weight management support

promoting local opportunities and community engagement

educating people about the benefits of healthy eating and physical activity further actions will be needed to improve public health spatial planning. The rest of this book aims to provide more information and advice on these.

Insider story 3.1: Insight from working with planners and public health teams to embed health in Essex, England

Laura Taylor-Green, head of public health and wellbeing at Essex County Council, shares her insight of joint working between planners and public health teams over the years. Laura had been working with planners and planning teams since 2015 to embed health into the planning work being done within local authorities in Essex. This started when she was asked to contribute to key projects that the planning teams were working on: the first was a strategic document on infrastructure needs over the next 20-plus years, where her input was needed to help understand the impacts on health infrastructure arising from population growth; the second was looking at integrating health and wellbeing principles into the design of new places through the local design guide.

Laura's contribution to the first project was providing an understanding of the complex health system and linking health service commissioners and providers. The second project involved being part of a wider stakeholder group providing guidance around the impact that places have on health and wellbeing, which then led to specific design principles being developed.

These two projects led to the start of embedding health into planning through the increased understanding of what public health does and what contribution public health could bring to place-based projects. Knowing that place influences health, wellbeing and health inequalities, mainly through the socio-economic influencers of health, such as education, income, employment, housing and transport, with the understanding that these are heavily influenced through place making, it became apparent very quickly that working together would bring real benefits to residents. At the same time that this agenda was being developed locally, the emphasis that national planning policy placed on health and wellbeing, and the influence of other bodies that promoted the need to bring health and planning together, such as the TCPA, PHE and NHS

England, had also begun to emerge more strongly, which helped support and drive forward her work.

Since these first two projects, there have since been local and national projects and activities, including strategy and policy development, training and skills support, input into planning applications, support on regeneration work, school design work, healthcare infrastructure, garden community development, HIAs, and quality design review work, which have led to the development of a charter and award specifically focused on healthy place making led by Chelmsford City Council. The variety of work, with so many organisations, highlights the interest in having public health input into planning matters. This was due to the understanding of the benefits in bringing planning and health together, not only in the county council, but also by many other organisations.

The scale and size of this agenda was significant, and the pace of work was fast. Therefore, building relationships with planners, supporting them in understanding this agenda and them supporting public health professionals was key. There were also several public health professionals who have planning within their portfolio, so linking into a wider network had been very useful and supportive.

Originally, her role sat in the public health team. As her work began to move more into the place agenda, in 2020, she was moved to sit within the department responsible for planning, transport, housing, economic growth and school infrastructure. The thinking behind this was that although her role had been able to support and influence decisions in the place department, by having her work directly within the teams responsible for the social determinants of health, there was a real opportunity to embed health in decision-making from the very start. This seemed to be the case, as she was part of the earliest conversations with people about health, health inequalities and what could be done to address these in the decisions being made, which Laura noted was really fantastic given that this work was just beginning.

Overall lesson

The most important thing that Laura learnt was understanding when it is possible to have influence. There was an enormous amount of potential benefit to health outcomes and health inequalities in addressing some of the key influencers of the socio-economic determinants of health through planning. This included looking at how people can work together to improve the physical environment so as to increase play and physical activity levels, increase active travel opportunities, increase employment access, address the food environment, and address the design of homes and spaces, which are all areas where health can get involved.

There are key stages in planning, so understanding when to be involved to provide support is important. The transferable skills in health, specifically around evidence reviews, population needs assessment and policy development, are all relevant to planning and can be very helpful to planning colleagues, especially when they are starting to develop their strategies and policies. Therefore, making links to the planning team to offer that support is a good first step.

The health impacts and potential health inequalities for specific population groups arising from planning are other areas where public health should get involved. Having this engagement early and speaking with planners on what they need from health also allows for this to be factored into the work programmes of public health teams. The planning process can run over many months or years, so having early sight of what capacity is needed in teams and what potential training or skills development may be required can then be considered.

Further information

Details about Essex's healthy development work are available at: www. essexdesignguide.co.uk/supplementary-guidance/livewell-developm ent-accreditation

PART II

Health, wellbeing and equity impacts

> Health in all policies ideally starts with the policy area (e.g. economic development policy or transport policy) not with a public health issue. This encourages thinking about the range of potential direct and indirect benefits/risks for health that can be created from that policy.
>
> LGA (2016)

It has been established that to significantly improve many of the health challenges facing communities today, there is a need to bring them to centre stage of the spatial planning system. This will ensure that the wider governance structures, policy frameworks and processes are clearly understood by both planning and public health professionals in a way that promotes joint working and collaboration. This part considers how health issues can be practically integrated with planning by outlining approaches and processes – beginning with the mainstreaming of an (HiAP) approach and then looking at the range of environmental impact and other health-related assessment requirements.

From a public health policy perspective, a key driver of enhancing health and wellbeing is to focus on embedding an HiAP approach. This can be achieved by using a range of methods and evidence-based assessment tools. Such tools can inform and assist decision-making in the formulation of planning and land-use policies, as well as the examination of the effects that specific urban development projects might have on health and wellbeing and the wider environment. From a spatial planning perspective, engaging with health and wellbeing stakeholders and policymakers can not only strengthen collaboration and long-term planning, but also enhance and strengthen elements of the spatial planning system to better incorporate core healthcare and public health policy issues in order to improve services, structures and sites.

This part provides an understanding of building health into a range of national, regional and local policies across a variety of sectors, including public health, healthcare services, planning, environmental sustainability, housing, transport and environmental health protection. It provides an overview of the challenges faced by those trying to bring a health dimension into planning and how these might be successfully addressed in a complex environment that might include legislators, developers and those who are commissioned or required to review actual impact assessments or plans and projects.

This part will enable readers to:

- understand the concept of HiAP and its importance and relevance in setting the wider operating context for implementing planning for health activities (see Chapter 4);
- understand how HIAs can enable the mobilisation of better health and address health inequalities in planning (see Chapter 5); and
- understand how health and HIA can be integrated into other impact assessments, the challenges in doing this, and how they can be overcome by drawing from a wealth of literature and guidance available to practitioners (see Chapter 6).

Part II key takeaways

- Embedding health considerations across all policy areas and decision-making systems can ensure multiple objectives can be achieved.
- Making improving health everybody's business can help stakeholders concurrently meet their respective social, economic, environmental and public health outcomes.
- Adopting HIAs can help improve the process and outcomes of spatial planning policies and decisions made on urban development projects.

- Adapting environmental impact and other health-related assessments to proportionally and systematically integrate health considerations can further improve process and outcomes.
- Recognising existing regulatory and practical challenges to integrating health considerations into impact assessment processes is the first step to overcoming them.

4

Health in All Policies

[HiAP is] an approach to public policies across sectors that systematically takes into account the health and health systems implications of decisions, seeks synergies and avoids harmful health impacts, in order to improve population health and health equity. It emphasizes the consequences of public policies on health determinants and inequalities, and aims to improve the accountability of policy-makers for health impacts at all levels of policy-making.

WHO (2014)

The aim of this chapter is to provide an overview of what HiAP is, set out its main tools and methods for implementation, and identify the key drivers for collaboration between spatial planning and health systems. It signposts the reader to useful resources that can assist and support officers to implement HiAP and its main tools.

What is HiAP?

HiAP has been developed by the WHO and, since the late 1970s, has been supported by governments across the world, such as Finland, Wales and South Australia (Leppo et al, 2013; Delany et al, 2016; Ståhl, 2018; WHO, 2018a). It was solidified at an international conference in 2010 and again in 2013, where the focus was on the approach and how it could be utilised and implemented in practice (WHO, 2010b, 2013b).

HiAP is an approach that seeks to improve population health and health equity by looking at public policies across all sectors. It does this by taking account of the health implications of decisions, seeking synergies and avoiding harmful health impacts and inequalities. In effect, it entails working collaboratively across sectors to inform and influence evidence-based decisions, so that any negative impacts on health and wellbeing are reduced, avoided or mitigated. It is preventative in nature and aims to address any social and health equity issues by focusing on the particular populations who will be affected by those decisions.

To communicate, implement and enable the concept of HiAP, engagement with colleagues in partner and other relevant organisations who are developing plans or strategies that are likely to affect health and wellbeing is essential. This involves working together to ensure these plans and strategies are shaped to improve health and wellbeing and reduce inequalities. It can include participating in partnership groups, collating and using health intelligence data and evidence, and leading or contributing to HIA or similar processes. For this to occur, sectors and systems need to speak to each other and create and develop solid and trustful long-term working relationships so that they can understand each other's terminology and perspectives. This can take time to evolve, both at a national and local level (WHO, 2018a), and many organisations and individuals carry it out subconsciously via consultation and informal partnership working.

HiAP is built on the foundations of six pillars and uses multidimensional methods and tools in its implementation (see Figure 4.1). At its core is a focus on intersectoral action and collaboration, and integrated working and involvement. Public participation is also a key aspect of HiAP drivers, and this assists private citizens' involvement in many of the decisions that affect their daily lives.

These actions can be applied by organisations and officers as a lens through which to implement, maximise or refine their approaches to mobilising HiAP as part of developing policies, implementing planning strategies and informing decisions on local plans and specific sites and developments. Table 4.1 articulates what these terms mean and some suggested ways of implementing them.

Figure 4.1: Interactions among HiAP pillars

HiAP approach					
Health, wellbeing, equity					
Pillar 1	Pillar 2	Pillar 3	Pillar 4	Pillar 5	Pillar 6
Governance	Planned action	Finances	Engagement and public involvement	Implementation, monitoring and evaluation	Capacity building

⬅️▬▬▬▬▬▬▬▬▬▬▬▬▬▬▬▬▬▬▬▬▬▬▬➡️

Table 4.1: HiAP pillars and implementation

Governance	Governance can provide the terms of reference for collective action (McQueen et al, 2012; WHO, 2018a). It can ensure that health, wellbeing and health equity are scoped into the process of collaboration and can prescribe the definition of health and wellbeing used, how it is to be fostered or governed, and how it can be integrated into decision-making (WHO, 2013b; Shankardass et al, 2015, 2018). Joint partnership or steering groups and regular engagement can provide a useful and beneficial framework for joint actions to implement HiAP.
Planned action	This can be short term by focusing on one particular aspect or work stream of mutual interest, for example, a new development or local plan, and by working together to achieve a tangible result and inform a specific decision to highlight the value of HiAP to partners (Ramirez-Rubio et al, 2019). It can also be long term and involve strategic planning to ensure that policy development and implementation are integrated and include a consideration of health, wellbeing and inequalities to strengthen spatial planning outcomes (Rogerson et al, 2020).
Finances	Intersectoral work, including joint funding bids, can ensure that resources are shared and used effectively. Research and practice has highlighted that dedicated staff and financial resources, for example, secondments and/or joint posts for public health-focused spatial planning officers or planning officers based in public health teams, can support the implementation of HiAP (Mundo et al, 2019; Rogerson et al, 2020).
Engagement and public involvement	Spatial plan requirements include the need to engage and consult with private citizens, communities and organisational stakeholders in decisions that affect them. Tools such as HIA or the Place Standard tool can assist in carrying out these aspects (Tamburrini et al, 2011; Public Health Scotland, 2017).

(continued)

Table 4.1: HiAP pillars and implementation (continued)

Implementation, monitoring and evaluation	Shared goals and outcomes, and joint funding and/or collaboration, between spatial planners and health teams can support health and wellbeing improvement and protection (WHO, 2013b). Setting targets for particular communities or groups can help to reduce inequalities and support implementation, statutory monitoring and reporting.
Capacity building	This can be achieved through developing organisational tools, processes, knowledge and experience. This can be carried out via training, practice-based learning (for example, HIA 'learning by doing' methods) and opportunities fostered through collaboration (Harris-Roxas and Harris, 2007; Freiler et al, 2013; WHO, 2013b; Green et al, 2020c).

Source: Cave et al (2016)

How does HiAP relate to spatial planning and public health systems?

Historically, there have been, and are, strong interconnecting relationships between public health and spatial planning systems, which means that there are benefits and synergies for both from adopting an HiAP approach (Harris et al, 2014). From a public health policy perspective, a key driver to enhancing health and wellbeing across sectors and multiple disciplines is to focus on HiAP, using a range of methods and tools to do this in order to drive health improvement and protection.

Planning departments, policies, plans and planning decisions can have a huge impact on health and wellbeing, and can have an enormous influence on the wider determinants of health (Geddes et al, 2011). They can: shape the environment we live in; make decisions about the siting and development of housing, green space, retail, leisure and employment facilities; and shape how we access and use these. Decisions can facilitate physical activity or access to fresh, quality food, or they can limit choices to do so, such as siting supermarkets in out-of-town retail parks to which local people have to drive versus local shops that are easy to walk or cycle to, or allocating green space for development or recreation and negotiating with developers about the extent of these. As NCDs, such as obesity, and associated ill health increase there is a need to make these connections to the built and natural environment more explicit.

HiAP can be achieved through working in partnership across sectors to deliver shared goals and have shared outcomes. Both systems are evidence based, and close collaboration can add to and support shared evidence bases. HiAP is nothing to be feared. Partnership working and collaboration, and involving and consulting with the public, are core aspects of both planning and public health functions. Doing so can foster better relationships, improve access to data and evidence, support regulatory and compulsory consultation processes, and, importantly, lead to the strengthening of sectors, policies, plans and projects, and to the implementation of healthy and strong policies, services and facilities, employment, and housing opportunities appropriate for the local community's needs. From a spatial planning perspective, engagement with health and wellbeing stakeholders and policymakers can not only strengthen collaboration and long-term planning, but also enhance the elements of the spatial planning system to be incorporated into healthcare and public health policymaking, thus improving services, structures and sites (Harris et al, 2014).

It must be stressed to, and understood by, public health professionals that health and wellbeing may not be the main focus of planners' activities, just as spatial planning is not the main focus of public health professionals' own activities. However, these do have a major influence on communities and individuals via the wider determinants of health outlined in Chapter 1, so this is key to collaborative working towards healthy and fairer community opportunities, services and facilities.

From a public health perspective, building health and wellbeing considerations and applying health-focused tools can support health policy decision-making, enable health improvement by mitigating for any negative implications for population groups and facilitate monitoring. It can also provide opportunities to provide and integrate health intelligence data and evidence to support and strengthen spatial planning decisions on the wider determinants of health, such as the built and natural environments, housing, green and blue infrastructure, transportation, air quality, and noise.

HiAP tools to strengthen planning and health and wellbeing action

HIA

HIA is a tool commonly advocated as a key vehicle through which to drive the concept of HiAP (WHO, 2015; Rogerson et al, 2020) and is a decision-informing tool that promotes cross-sector collaboration (Green et al, 2021a). HIA is defined as 'a combination of procedures, methods and tools by which a policy, intervention or service may be judged as to its potential effects on the health of a population, and the distribution of those effects within a population' (ECHP, 1999; WHO, 2021b). It is an evidence-based practical, systematic and yet flexible tool through which policymakers can establish whether their work could have an impact on the population and, if so, how this will affect them (that is, positive, negative or unintended negative impacts). It does this through the lens of the social determinants of health, for example, social, community, environmental or economic impacts, and identifies which particular groups will be affected, for example, older people, those on low incomes and so on.

HIA is also a valuable tool because it provides practical and realistic recommendations for action to maximise any positive impacts or opportunities, and mitigate any negative or unintended negative impacts. HIA also has a monitoring stage that can seamlessly be included in annual monitoring plans. HIA and the process is described in more detail in Chapter 5.

Health lens analysis

The health lens analysis process builds on HIA methodology. It was developed in South Australia and can also be utilised to support HiAP (Van Eyk et al, 2017) and adapted to the operational culture and policies of each partner agency. As a consequence, the methodology employed for a health lens is modified for each target area. Evaluation is an essential component of the HiAP process, and it is built into each individual health lens.

The emerging methodology for health lens analysis underpinning its effectiveness and ability to deliver outcomes that are mutually beneficial to all parties consists of the following steps:

1. Engage: establishing and maintaining strong collaborative relationships with other sectors to determine an agreed policy focus.
2. Gather evidence: establishing impacts between health and the policy area under focus, and identifying evidence-based solutions or policy options.
3. Generate: producing a set of policy recommendations and a final report that are jointly owned by all partner agencies.
4. Navigate: helping to steer recommendations through the decision-making process.
5. Evaluate: determining the effectiveness of the health lens.

Opportunities and synergies to mobilise HiAP in planning for health

There are many opportunities for joint working to inform decision-making and planning, which can generate win–win situations (see Table 4.2):

- *Policies, strategies and plans* for national, regional and local spatial and health services, for example: national planning and development frameworks; sustainable development or public health legislation; and local policies for green and blue space, hot-food takeaways, economic development and employment, and active transport and travel (Ramirez-Rubio et al, 2019; Rogerson et al, 2020).
- *Projects*, including national and local new or extended infrastructure projects, for example, new roads, new rail lines, regenerating town and other centres, and environmental, green and climate-focused projects.
- *Proposed or extended development sites*, including housing, employment, infrastructure sites like healthcare services sites, estates, and retail sites.

There are also many examples of collaborative working across the world between health and spatial planning (Harris et al,

Table 4.2: Examples of win–win situations for planning for health

	Spatial planning	Public health and healthcare
Strengthen plans and policies for the whole community	✓	✓
Take a preventative approach by mitigating any detrimental impacts or risks	✓	✓
Develop infrastructure, services, sites and facilities appropriate and fit for local needs and the wellbeing of everyone in a community or place	✓	✓
Involve and consult with key stakeholders, including communities and the general public	✓	✓
Identify, use, develop and generate data, evidence and knowledge bases for decision-making	✓	✓

2014; Ramirez-Rubio et al, 2019; Rogerson et al, 2020). Some of these are also highlighted in the 'insider stories' contained in this book, which provide some real-world successful collaborative examples. Examples can be found in the work carried out by PHE, Public Health Wales and local authorities.

While there are huge opportunities to build an HiAP approach into spatial planning policies, plans and supportive tools, particularly in the UK (PHE, 2020b; Green et al, 2021a; Johnson and Green, 2021; Public Health Scotland, 2021), it should be noted that there are challenges to wider integrated working (Ramirez-Rubio et al, 2019). These can include, for example, the lack of: shared data and evidence; training, resources and capacity; and awareness of health and a plethora of other mandatory assessments, such as strategic environmental assessments (SEAs) and integrated impact assessments (IIAs), which may include a consideration of health, but can dilute the health and equity focus (Mundo et al, 2019; Rogerson et al, 2020; Green et al, 2021a).

Potential actions

Practitioners and their organisations can think through and develop how they implement HiAP by building on existing work that has taken place across their context or internationally. Examples of actions can include:

- accessing any information, advice, guidance or support provided by public health organisations and institutions, HIA units, and spatial planning and health teams in their locality or nation;
- directly engaging with spatial planning, healthcare services or public health partners and their officers to discuss potential collaboration (have a current or proposed plan, policy, project or development that you could highlight that could tentatively focus discussion, or look to identify mutual work streams and the future opportunities/challenges and benefits for both);
- exploring shared resources and joint capacity-building programmes;
- utilising levers, such as national or local spatial planning frameworks and documents, or healthy public policy-focused laws, strategies or plans; and
- developing an understanding of the terminology and existing frameworks that each sector uses, and the contexts in which they are used (it is helpful to map out and scope the language and frameworks at the start, and to identify any individuals, resources or organisations that can help practitioners 'translate' the system and language, as organisations will need to consider the most useful and relevant terminology for their own policy and political context, and utilise any common language that is already used in or for joint working).

The Scottish Place Standard tool

Developed in Scotland, the Place Standard tool enables communities, public agencies, voluntary groups and others to find those aspects of a place that need to be targeted to improve people's health, wellbeing and quality of life. It is a way of assessing places, be they well established, changing or being planned, and the tool can be useful to aid or initiate discussions about the physical elements of a place or space, and how these can be maximised to benefit the community and the individuals who work, visit and reside there. Understanding the existing strengths and weaknesses of a place can enable targeted action to improve the population's lives and reduce inequalities. (For more information, see: www.healthscotland.scot/health-inequalities/impact-of-social-and-physical-environments/place/the-place-standard-tool)

Concluding statement

HiAP is a concept that many planners and public health or healthcare representatives and officers can implement when they work in collaboration or consult with each other. By formalising ways of working, they can strengthen the delivery of policies, plans and sites to the communities that they serve, and enable shared planning and health outcomes.

By enabling discussions, explaining the terminology and aims, and outlining positions at the start of the process, there is nothing to be feared on either side; indeed, this can lead to arrangements that are more formal and the creation of long-term fruitful relationships and understanding. However, for HiAP to be of benefit, it must have practical support – human and financial resources – to create or use supportive systems and resources, such as joint evidence bases or HIA toolkits like the highlighted examples from Wales in Chapter 5.

Insider story 4.1: Integrating health and health equity into local government in Australia

Associate Professor Fiona Haigh, Manager of the HIA Support Unit, Centre for Primary Health Care and Equity at the University of New South Wales, Australia, reflects on integrating health and planning in Wollondilly. Wollondilly Shire is a peri-urban area located on the south-western fringe of Greater Sydney. The area provides a transition between the outer edges of the major city of Sydney and regional New South Wales, and is characterised by a mix of rural towns, villages, agriculture and bushlands. Its current population of around 51,000 is set to almost double over the next 20 years, with two designated growth areas to provide housing for Sydney.

Health services in Australia have a mandated role to promote, protect and maintain the health of residents. However, most of what determines health lies outside of the direct control of health services and the health system. Local governments are uniquely positioned to address the social determinants of health and existing health inequities in communities through shaping land development and usage. Traditionally, local health services have engaged with local government through making formal submissions to councils on their strategic documents and major developments. However, over the years, Population Health, a unit within the South Western Sydney Local Health District (SWSLHD), identified that developing closer partnerships with local government could assist with addressing the social determinants of health and began to look for ways to do this.

This work began in 2013, when the health service approached Wollondilly Shire Council (WSC) to undertake an HIA as part of an HIA 'learning by doing' training model. This involved forming a team with representatives from the health service and WSC to work together on an HIA of a proposed new town. After completion of the HIA, senior management from both organisations met to discuss ways to build on the HIA and collaboratively work together on projects, with the aim of incorporating health considerations into council planning processes. This began a multi-year process of engagement between a local government, local health services and an academic research centre (the Centre for Health Equity Research, Training and Evaluation) focused on a series of joint projects. The first project aimed to develop a shared understanding of land-use planning processes and to identify opportunities for the consideration of health within those processes. The project involved key informant interviews, along with participant observation of select planning meetings and a document review of a number of state and local land-use planning documents. This was supplemented by a literature review to identify existing tools and strategies that could be used to integrate health into land-use planning.

What happened?

Three key actions were implemented as a result of the project findings. A health vision was incorporated into the community strategic plan (CSP). This is the highest level of strategic planning undertaken by a local council and is used by council and other agencies and stakeholders to guide policy and service delivery. A co-funded (SWSLHD and WSC) senior strategic health planner post was created, and a health assessment protocol for land-use and strategic planning was developed. The protocol utilises tools and processes that fit the WSC context, and considers local government environment and council processes. This has now led to the development of health and social impact assessment policy and guidelines.

The relationship between the partners was also formalised into the Health and Planning Working Group, which meets regularly. The model of co-funded local government and health positions has been rolled out to two other local government areas, with more roles being developed. As well as the concrete outcomes of policies, tools and joint positions, an evaluation of the programme of work identified such benefits as: increased levels of understanding of the relationship between the work of local government and the determinants of health; the increased currency of health and health equity as an idea; improved trust between partners; and improved understanding of how partners can work together.

What is the overall observable lesson?

Beginning the process by carrying out an HIA was purposeful. There was already an understanding that an HIA is a powerful way of developing relationships between different sectors and a shared understanding of determinants of health and health equity.

Using a 'learning by doing' approach works well because having a real-life HIA to focus on makes the learning process meaningful and requires high-level buy-in that creates a supportive environment. Working together on a shared project over time while learning together built trust and relationships between the health service and WSC staff. This created support for the next stage of the project, which involved an in-depth process of identifying barriers and opportunities within WSC planning and policymaking processes. These included such issues as: planners viewing perceived unnecessary standards as a risk to development processes; regulatory constraints and developer pressures, meaning that planners were disinclined to go beyond minimum standards to require healthy developments; and health needing to be integrated at multiple levels within the council to create a supportive environment for change.

The follow-on project was important, in that it focused on understanding the local context so that the recommendations developed were fit for purpose and feasible. Relevant theory-based approaches were drawn upon by viewing WSC as a complex adaptive system and utilising policy, learning and implementation science theories to help explain how to create organisational change. The tools that were developed look very similar to other existing health in planning tools, but they could not have been implemented without having had a process of creating a supportive environment and building capacity.

Further information

Details of Wollondilly's health and planning work are available at: www. healthyactivebydesign.com.au/case-studies/health-and-planning-in-wollondilly

5

Health Impact Assessment in planning

> Health Impact Assessment (HIA) makes a valuable contribution towards plan making. It may be useful when proposing or making decisions on new development ... Evidence on health impacts can help the planning system develop stronger and more coherent approaches towards maximising health and well-being.
>
> Welsh Government (2021a)

This chapter outlines the process of an HIA, the roles carried out in an HIA, how it can be used as a beneficial and proportional process to support effective public health spatial planning and decision-making, and its integration in practice.

What is an HIA?

An HIA is a flexible and systematic tool that can be applied to effectively implement HiAP approaches at local, national and regional levels. It considers in an explicit and effective way the populations impacted by development or spatial planning policy and plans, and can address and help to discuss and mitigate any issues before they arise. HIA is defined as 'a combination of procedures, methods and tools by which a policy, intervention or service may be judged as to its potential effects on the health of a population, and the distribution of those effects within a population' (ECHP, 1999). Underpinned by the WHO's holistic definition of health and wellbeing, it uses the social determinants of health as a lens through which to identify health impacts (WHO, 1946).

The HIA process

As a process, HIA is systematic and scalable, which allows health and wellbeing to be considered in all policy sectors in a proportionate way. The process explicitly raises awareness of wellbeing and inequalities among policy and decision-makers and officers (Parry and Scully, 2003; Simpson et al, 2005; Winkler et al, 2021), and is recommended by the WHO as an important method with which to drive and apply HiAP to support healthy public policymaking (WHO, 2014). HIA is explicitly tied to HiAP, as it can enable collaboration across sectors to influence and inform decision-making processes, identifies positive and negative impacts on the population, and makes recommendations to mitigate and avoid them (Winkler et al, 2013). However, previous evidence acknowledges that there can be both benefits and challenges attached to the use of HIA (Huang, 2012; Tamburrini et al, 2011; Winkler et al, 2021).

The process uses the determinants of health as a lens through which to assess the impact of policies, plans or projects. It follows a broad mixed-methods approach to HIA, considers the potential positive and the negative (and unintended negative) impacts across the breadth of determinants, and focuses on the impact on health equity and vulnerable populations, for example, women, children and young people, or older people. It does this via two checklists that focus on population groups and the wider determinants of health and wellbeing (Green et al, 2020d; WHIASU, 2021). The HIA process also directly involves organisations, institutions, public bodies and communities (and their representatives) that could, or will, be affected by the policy or plan under assessment, or that have an interest in it (Winkler et al, 2021; Green et al, 2021a).

HIA is a five-step process, consisting of screening, scoping, appraisal of the evidence, recommedations and reporting, and review and reflection (including monitoring and evaluation) (Green et al, 2021a). Figure 5.1 depicts the process to be

Figure 5.1: The HIA process

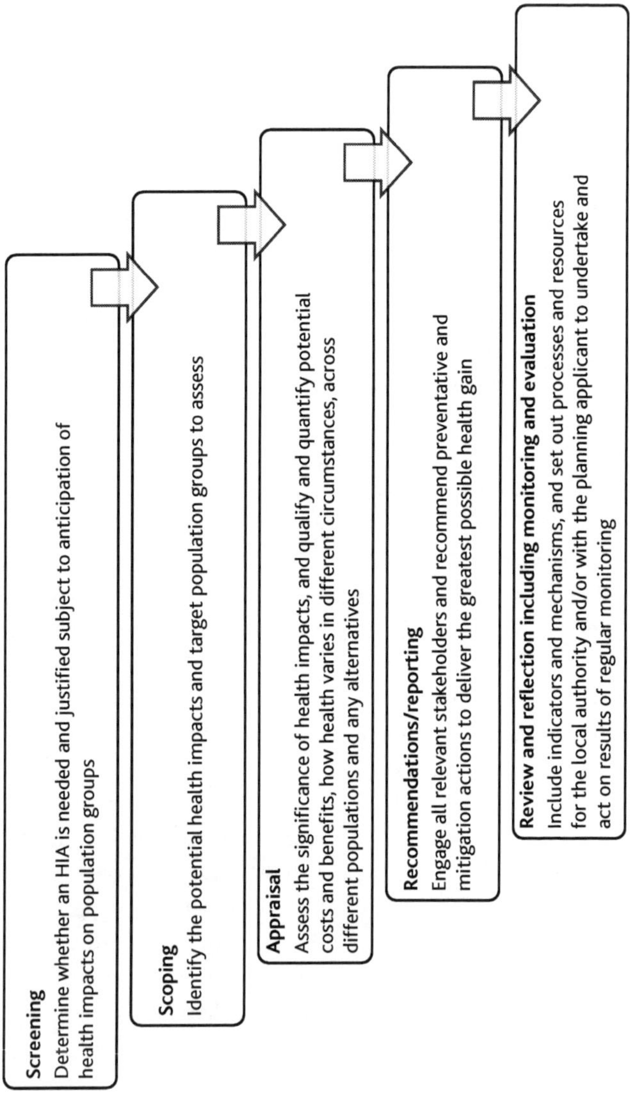

Screening
Determine whether an HIA is needed and justified subject to anticipation of health impacts on population groups

Scoping
Identify the potential health impacts and target population groups to assess

Appraisal
Assess the significance of health impacts, and qualify and quantify potential costs and benefits, how health varies in different circumstances, across different populations and any alternatives

Recommendations/reporting
Engage all relevant stakeholders and recommend preventative and mitigation actions to deliver the greatest possible health gain

Review and reflection including monitoring and evaluation
Include indicators and mechanisms, and set out processes and resources for the local authority and/or with the planning applicant to undertake and act on results of regular monitoring

followed. While some may regard it as a linear process, HIAs are most useful and effective when the process is iterative and can be adapted to particular timescales and circumstances. The process is not detailed in this chapter, but explained comprehensively in many of the HIA guides available across the world (Harris et al, 2007; WHIASU, 2012; Pyper et al, 2021; SOPHIA, 2021).

Perspectives on HIA

There are two primary perspectives that inform the practice of HIA (Kemm, 2003). First, there is the 'tight' HIA, which tends to be epidemiologically focused – mainly on quantifiable and physical health impacts, such as air quality, emissions, noise levels and visual impacts. This perspective was developed out of environmental impact assessment (EIA) (Birley et al, 1998; Wismar et al, 2007; Cave et al, 2021).

Second, there is the 'broad' HIA, which: is more sociological in nature; uses a social and holistic definition of health; acknowledges that there are different theories of change and health impact; addresses the complex nature of the contexts to which proposals refer; has a broader understanding of what constitutes knowledge and evidence; and may include the accounts and perspectives of lay communities (Tamburrini et al, 2011; Green et al, 2020b; WHO, 2021b). A consideration of health inequalities and equity should be an integral component of any HIA (Kemm et al, 2004; Winkler et al, 2021). In nation states that have a legislative requirement for HIA and a focus on equity, for example, in Wales, all HIAs must systematically consider inequalities between, and the impacts on, a range of population groups, and assess the extent and distribution of these impacts (WHIASU, 2012; Green et al, 2021a). These groups can, for example, include older people, children and young people, and those who suffer from chronic conditions or are geographically isolated. HIA is also based on a number of key principles and values – these include equity, robustness, openness, transparency, ethical use of evidence, participation, sustainability and democracy.

There is no 'right' or 'wrong' way to carry out an HIA, but the approach taken needs to be carefully scoped and clearly articulated as to why a specific approach was taken. A robust, useful and holistic HIA will use mixed qualitative and quantitative methods, using the theories, concepts and methods of sociology, epidemiology and other disciplines as necessary, with an equal importance attached to democracy and scientific credibility.

Typologies of HIA

Types of HIA in spatial planning

There are three main types of HIA, and they can embrace differing perspectives and policy levels:

- Prospective HIA: conducted at the start of the development of a project, proposal or plan. Anticipates impact.
- Concurrent HIA: runs alongside the implementation of the project (or policy). Captures evidence as it emerges and can inform and influence changes to plans or policies as they are implemented and reviewed at nominated times.
- Retrospective HIA: assesses the effect of an existing project or policy, and can be used as an evaluation and review tool. Retrospective assessments can be carried out on unexpected or unanticipated plans and unique events, such as Brexit. They capture existing published evidence and can discuss the effect of implementation with key stakeholders as way of learning lessons and informing any future similar events.

HIA is routinely promoted as providing most value when utilised prospectively during the development of a proposal (Parry and Stevens, 2001). The process should be activated late enough in a proposal's development to be clear about its nature and purpose, but early enough to be able to influence its design and/ or implementation. However, there are some clear examples of HIAs carried out in real time as a policy or plan is being implemented that have provided evidence and information for policy and decision-makers and planners (Kögel et al, 2020; Green et al, 2021a), and these have highlighted the benefits of these approaches – particularly in emergency situations or unique events, where decisions have been taken at speed.

Within any of the aforementioned types, an HIA can also take several different forms, depending on the focus and the time and resources available: desktop, rapid (including a participatory workshop) or comprehensive (Birley, 2011). In practice, the most commonly used is a rapid HIA (Chilaka, 2010). Often, any particular HIA may fit in between two of these forms, as the approach taken will be determined by the nature of the proposal, the timescales involved and the human, organisational and financial resources available to undertake the process.

Forms of HIAs

- A *desktop HIA* exercise can take hours or a day, and can encompass a small number of stakeholders to utilise existing knowledge and evidence to assess a proposal, policy or plan.
- A *rapid (including participatory) HIA* can take days or weeks and usually includes the establishment of a small steering group and a participatory workshop – in which there is a brief investigation of the health impacts on the local population and the gathering of knowledge and further evidence from a number of key stakeholders. This type of HIA also includes a short literature review of quantitative and qualitative evidence, health intelligence, and other demographic data to form a better understanding of the impacts.
- A *comprehensive HIA* is more in-depth and can take several weeks or months to complete. Comprehensive HIAs are not completed as frequently as desktop or rapid HIAs, which can be attributed to the fact that they can be time and resource intensive and require knowledge of the policy context and more wide-ranging evidence obtained via literature searches, the collection of primary quantitative and qualitative data (such as interviews or workshops), and more focused health intelligence and demographic statistics.

Characterisation of impact

There are a variety of ways in which the potential impacts may be described (Table 5.1). Where possible, the following impacts should be assessed:

Table 5.1: Terminology: characterisation of impact

Positive – impacts that improve or maintain health status

Negative – impacts that diminish health status

Confirmed – actual direct evidence in existence

Probable – more likely to happen than not, direct evidence but from limited sources

Possible – may or may not happen

Significant – sufficiently great or important to be worthy of attention, noteworthy

Moderate – average in intensity quality or degree

Minimal – of a minimum amount, quantity or degree, negligible

S = short term – less than one year

SM = short to medium term – one to three years

ML = medium to long term – three to five or 10 years

L = 10 or more years

- Nature of the impact: how will the proposal affect health, and will the impact be positive or negative? Will it be direct or indirect, that is, via a direct pathway or as an associated impact?
- Likelihood of the impact: is the likelihood of the impact of the proposal confirmed, probable or possible?
- Scale and significance of the impact: what proportion of the population is likely to be affected? How significant, moderate or minimal will the impact be (that is, will it cause mild ill health, improve wellbeing or lead to deaths)?
- Timing of the impact: will the impact be in the short, medium or long term? In some instances, the short-term risks to health may be worth the long-term benefits.
- Distribution of the effects: will the proposal affect different groups of people in different ways? A proposal that is likely to benefit one section of the population, for example, older people, may not benefit others, for example, children and young people. The assessment will identify the ways in which members of the least healthy or most vulnerable populations could be helped. This can be an important contribution to reducing the health inequalities that exist in some communities.

What evidence is acceptable?

HIA utilises both qualitative and quantitative types of evidence. Where an estimation of the size of an impact can be measured, for instance, when estimating the increase of airborne particulates due to changes in traffic variations and the resultant impact on the health and wellbeing of nearby communities, then quantitative methods may be most appropriate or modelling techniques can be used to project and anticipate impact.

However, some potential health impacts are not easy to measure, but they may be equally or more important in terms of their impact on population health. Shutting a community facility, such as a library, for example, can have a range of impacts. These impacts can manifest themselves in myriad ways, which can only be assessed through more qualitative methods that explore people's feelings, experiences or perspectives. 'Improving the use of evidence in health impact assessment' (Mindell et al, 2010) provides useful information to support HIA practitioners when assessing the quality and type of evidence included in HIAs. The Wales Health Impact Assessment Support Unit (WHIASU) and Ben Cave Associates have also published critical quality assurance review frameworks for HIA that focus on the process, the evidence used, the participation and contributions, and the report itself (Fredsgaard et al, 2009; Green et al, 2019).

The roles in HIA

There are several different roles in play when an HIA is commissioned, carried out and reviewed. HIAs can be carried out or reviewed by anyone who can follow the process outlined in a recognised guide (Harris et al, 2007; Fredsgaard et al, 2009; WHIASU, 2012; Pyper et al, 2021). This includes individuals, private and public organisations like local government or health agencies, developers, or communities (Elliott and Williams, 2008, Winkler et al, 2021). There is a misapprehension within some organisations that an HIA will be carried out by an individual. However, this is not good practice. In reality, HIA should be a collective and multidisciplinary process, with a nominated lead and a variety of contributors – ranging from a nominated lead who understands the process and can use the tools available, to health intelligence and data leads who can provide evidence, to administrators who can support the process in practice, set up meetings and so on, through to reviewers who can quality-assure the report. This approach is similar to multidisciplinary teams who carry out an SEA and EIA. WHIASU published an HIA training and capacity-building framework that outlined relevant roles and their component parts (Edmonds et al, 2019), as summarised in Table 5.2.

Table 5.2 makes it explicit which role can be carried out as part of an HIA and individuals' contribution. But what about the specific sector's team, department or organisation, and their roles? Table 5.3 depicts the roles of key stakeholders in commissioning,

Table 5.2: Different roles of professionals in the HIA process

Role	Definition
Advocate/system leader	Advocates for HiAP, champions the use of HIA, provides leadership and identifies opportunities to use HIA.
Authoriser	Commissions and/or allocates resources to HIA and integrates HiAP into organisational structures and work plans. Holds overall ownership and accountability for HIAs that they authorise or commission.
Stakeholder	Participates in an HIA as a key stakeholder, community member, lay representative and so on.
Contributor	Contributes to an HIA with a particular skill set or knowledge.
Reviewer	Carries out quality assurance reviews, monitoring and evaluation of HIAs. Provides clear feedback to commissioners and decision-makers.
Lead HIA practitioner (intermediate) – screening and desktop HIAs	Leads the planning, design, delivery and evaluation of desktop HIAs or HIA screening focused on a discrete project, policy or service area. Ensures that the HIA process follows guidance and benchmarks for high-quality HIAs.
Lead HIA practitioner (advanced) – comprehensive, complex and participatory HIAs	Leads the planning, design, delivery and evaluation of participatory, complex, contentious and/or large-scale comprehensive HIAs. Ensures that the HIA process follows guidance and benchmarks for high-quality HIAs.

Table 5.3: Stakeholder roles in HIA

	Spatial planners	Public health officers	Communities and society	Developers	Commissioned consultants
Advocate	✓	✓	✓	✓	✓
Authoriser/ commissioner	✓	✓		✓	
Lead HIA practitioner (intermediate)	✓	✓			✓
Lead HIA practitioner (advanced)	✓	✓			✓
Stakeholder	✓	✓	✓	✓	
Contributor	✓	✓	✓	✓	
Reviewer – quality assurance	✓	✓	✓	✓	✓

carrying out and reviewing HIAs, and demonstrates that there are a wide range of possible leads, contributors and reviewers within HIA practice. However, it is not essential that one organisation or team will have to fill every role, and these may be interchangeable based on the scope, scale, nature and significance of each HIA carried out.

For example, spatial planners may commission an HIA, contribute to it as a stakeholder or sit on a steering group setting the scope and then either review it or ask local public health officers to do so. A housing developer may commission an HIA but then let those commissioned to carry out the work and only review it or interrogate it at the end of the process, prior to submission for planning permission.

It must be stressed that carrying out a fit-for-purpose, quality HIA is not, and should not be, a one-person task. HIAs need to be proportionate and manageable within the resources that are available, but that should not limit wider contributions or interaction with key stakeholders. A participatory interactive workshop (either virtual or in person) can be a time-efficient and resource-effective method of engaging with stakeholders and collecting evidence.

Using HIAs to inform the planning process

Conducting an HIA within the planning, regeneration and housing sectors can confer considerable benefits, and contribute to healthy public policy and urban and rural planning. HIA will not only assess the potential positive and negative impacts, but also highlight any potential improvements that could be made to maximise health and wellbeing, and identify and mitigate any detrimental impacts or unintended consequences. HIA can make more explicit the links between land use and associated planning decisions, the way that we live, and the key health and wellbeing issues today, including obesity, lack of physical activity and the associated risk factors and illnesses.

It directly involves key local organisational and community stakeholders, as well as those who have local knowledge and understanding of how the project, plan or proposal will have a direct and indirect impact on local populations (Haigh et al, 2015; Winkler et al, 2021). An HIA can give context to a decision or plan. This includes how a community interacts with its physical and built environment, and can facilitate physical health promotion and health improvement by encouraging cycle paths, pedestrian-friendly towns, more active travel, open and green space allocation for recreation and sport, and access to the growth and purchase of fresh and affordable food in local plans and housing developments.

Carrying out HIAs has benefits not only for the policy and plan makers, but also for the developers, public health, the environment and, most importantly, the communities that are affected by these. Despite this, and until recently, not all local authorities have reflected the importance of health in planning decisions, such as in relation to green spaces, recreational areas or person-centred built environments. This is now changing as obesity and associated ill health increases, awareness of the implications of spatial planning in relation to such emergencies as COVID-19 increases and supportive resources and reviews are published (PHE, 2018; Green et al, 2021a; Winkler et al, 2021).

Benefits and challenges to the use of HIA in spatial planning

There are many benefits to requiring and carrying out an HIA to assess the impacts of spatial planning policies, plans and development projects (Tamburrini et al, 2011; Cave et al, 2020; Green et al, 2021a; Winkler et al, 2021). These include:

- increasing awareness across sectors of how planning could impact on health and wellbeing and inequalities;
- involving the key stakeholders who may be affected by, or have an interest in, the plan and the process by bringing them together as part of workshops or focus groups in an open way to discuss issues of concern;
- coordinating action between sectors to protect health and societal wellbeing;
- promoting evidence-based planning and decision-making; and
- giving a clearer view of what is being planned and what impact there might be on the community in the short, medium and long term.

HIAs should be an integral component in assessing the benefits and harms of planning-related topics. Ideally, they should be conducted *prior* to any proposals being formulated, integrated throughout the development of a plan or development, or at specific consultation junctures, for example, in the UK, as part of the preferred strategy stage of local development plans (LDPs). The evidence-based findings and recommendations should be used within the planning and/or development process to address and mitigate any potential negative impacts or unintended negative impacts, but they can also be used as a platform to maximise any positive impacts or opportunities (see Table 5.4).

Involving the community is an integral aspect of an HIA process (Mahoney et al, 2007; Elliott and Williams, 2008; Chadderton et al, 2013; Green et al, 2021a; Winkler et al, 2021) and can be used to complement and inform robust research and other evidence and data. This is when the appraisal of evidence is very beneficial in HIA, as it provides a holistic and evidence-based understanding of how any plans or policies may

Table 5.4: Benefits of HIA

Benefit	Spatial planners	Public health officers	Communities and society	Developers
Strengthen and improve policies, plans and developments by mitigating negative and unintended negative impacts, and maximising positive impacts and opportunities	✓	✓	✓	✓
Develop health, wellbeing and equity-focused plans and developments that are desirable, viable and fit for local purposes	✓	✓	✓	✓
Engage key stakeholders in a systematic and focused method	✓	✓	✓	✓
Identify key local knowledge and evidence	✓	✓	✓	✓
Inform decisions, including midterm reviews that provide opportunities to change plans and policies based on emerging evidence, and to learn from the implementation of these to date	✓	✓		✓
Identify opportunities for further integration and collaboration between sectors, and to connect key stakeholders to each other	✓	✓		✓
Standalone HIAs can add value to other impact assessment processes that are being, or have been, carried out	✓	✓	✓	✓

play out. The development of shared evidence bases and shared knowledge between public health and local or national planners is particularly helpful to strengthen both plans and population health, and can lead to shared outcomes and public benefit (TCPA and WHIASU, 2016; Johnson and Green, 2021).

However, there can be several challenges to the implementation of HIA. While the definition of HIA is generally agreed upon, complicating matters is the fact that countries have different legislative/regulatory frameworks and public health and planning systems that have differing foci and priorities. As such, HIAs must be designed within these contexts and their constraints, and should be proportionate yet robust. As previously referred to, there are many guides on how to undertake HIAs (Harris et al, 2007; WHIASU, 2012; Douglas, 2019; WHIASU, 2021; WHO, 2021b) and focused critical appraisal tools that can help to ensure the process is of sufficient quality (Fredsgaard et al, 2009; Green et al, 2017).

In terms of carrying out HIAs on a plan or policy, there may be no or little capacity to carry out an HIA in an organisation or planning authority. However, there is guidance that describes how HIAs can be carried out 'in-house' in a proportionate and time-effective and efficient way (PHE, 2020b; Cave et al, 2021, Green et al, 2021a; Johnson and Green, 2021). This lack of capacity and capability to undertake HIAs in local planning teams (which could also be reflected in any local or national public health teams who could assist them), has led to an increased growth in HIA consultants and health-focused leads at environmental consultancies. In the main, due to the consultancies they sit in, the latter tend to have a primary focus on environmental health determinants only, rather than a focus on the wider determinants of health and health inequalities.

Issues around the financing of, capacity building for and resourcing of HIAs to be carried out can create situations in which those with particular interests (for example, developers and extraction industries) can, and do, fund HIAs or elements of an HIA. This is more routinely as part of a statutory obligation to conduct an EIA (Harris et al, 2014; Cave et al, 2020). Therefore, if an HIA is commissioned, the likelihood is that the developer will pay for it and any HIA will be undertaken alongside their statutory obligation to conduct an EIA. Clearly, this situation could be construed as a conflict of interest by key stakeholders, such as local communities, and compromise the study. This can lead to a distrust of any findings or recommendations by public health practitioners and citizens, particularly regarding planning decisions, and can be challenging to surmount.

Additionally, an obstacle to overcome can be how to manage a community's expectations of what an HIA can and cannot achieve and to minimise jargon. HIA is a balanced process that assesses both positive and negative impacts, and the evidence for both must be transparently published. Therefore, the aims and objectives of any HIA must be established and communicated from the outset, which requires the involvement of or consultation with stakeholders, such as local public health teams, at the start of the planning process, and ensuring that their voices are heard and acted upon. The HIA should be used as a transparent vehicle to gather data and evidence of all types to use in and to support planning decision and policymaking processes while strengthening their outcomes (Table 5.5).

Concluding statement

This chapter has focused on HIA in more general terms and in relation to its application in spatial planning. HIAs can also be used for a wide range of policies, plans and development initiatives in a wide range of specific sectors. These include housing, commercial and retail, place making, the natural environment (including creating green and blue space), regeneration, and transport.

An HIA is a flexible, systematic and scalable tool. It can be applied to a variety of plans, policies and development projects in spatial planning. It can provide a balanced, wide-ranging, evidence-based overview of the positive impacts and good practice derived from these plans and projects, while also identifying negative or unintended negative impacts for communities and particular population groups. This allows for constructive conversations to enhance opportunities or mitigate negative impacts within planning processes in a proportionate and practical way.

Table 5.5: Strategic considerations in maximising the application of HIAs in planning policy development: Wales example

	Key points	
HIAs and planning policy	Why undertake an HIA?	✓ Ensure robust evidence base for health and wellbeing ✓ Identify local health needs/issues directly with relevant stakeholders in a participatory manner ✓ Ensure policies reflect appropriate local community needs ✓ Development plan supports healthy and sustainable communities
	Who should undertake an HIA?	✓ Local planning authority ✓ In-house (consider local organisational involvement) ✓ External consultants
	When should HIA be undertaken?	✓ At an early stage ✓ Evidence gathering ✓ Issues and options ✓ Preferred strategy (as part of consultation to maximise benefits) ✓ Deposit stage
	What type of HIA should be undertaken?	LDP (new and review) or supplementary planning document ✓ Rapid participatory HIA
	How should HIA be undertaken?	There are two ways of undertaking HIA ✓ Standalone assessment ✓ Integration within the wider sustainability appraisal process
	What is the benefit of an HIA?	✓ Additional qualitative and quantitative evidence provided to add to existing base ✓ Fits into all consultation stages as a participatory process ✓ Improved links to such policy areas and sectors as public health and wellbeing agendas ✓ Increased mutual understanding among public health practitioners and planning professionals ✓ Demonstrable understanding, accountability and consideration of the impact of planning on the health and wellbeing of the local population/community

Source: Green et al (2021a)

6

Health in other impact assessments

> Health is an increasingly important component
> in many *ex-ante* decision-making support impact
> assessment (IA) instruments ... This continues to be
> a developing agenda which brings new actors and
> new perspectives into established IA systems.
>
> Fischer and Cave (2018, p 1)

Health and its meaning

'Health' can be described and interpreted in different ways and
mean different things to different individuals, communities and
practitioners, dependent on their local context, knowledge,
practice and beliefs (Tamm, 1993; Larson, 1999). Health can
be categorised as:

- *A medical model*: this focuses on the physical body itself and
  disease, illness and death. The body is something to be
  healed and measured in a negative way (Stokes et al, 1982).
  Population health would be presented as statistics, for example,
  levels of disease or life expectancy rates.
- *A holistic model*: this focuses on both physical and mental health
  and wellbeing (WHO, 1946). It views health as something that
  can be measured both positively and negatively. However, the
  concept of wellbeing can be difficult to capture compared to
  rates of disease, which are more readily available. Population
  health would be measured through statistics and data, such

as levels of disease and life expectancy rates, and wellbeing through proxy indicators, such as levels of physical activity, and dietary indicators, such as the amount of fresh fruit or vegetables eaten per day.

• *A wellness model*: the WHO definition was further expanded in the 1986 Ottawa Charter for Health Promotion, which focused on the extent to which an individual or group is able to attain their aspirations and needs, and to adapt or be resilient in the context of their environment. It states: 'health is a resource for everyday life, not the objective of living; it is a positive concept, emphasizing social and personal resources, as well as physical capacities' (WHO, 1986, p 1). It views health as something that can be measured both positively and negatively. However, the concept of wellbeing can be difficult to capture compared to rates of disease, which are more readily available (University of Ottawa, 2021). Population health would be measured through statistics and data, for example, levels of disease and life expectancy rates. Wellbeing would be measured through proxy indicators, such as levels of physical activity, and dietary indicators, such as the amount of fresh fruit or vegetables eaten per day, or how happy someone is.

• *An environmental model*: this focuses on physical health risk and the negative effects resulting from the interaction with a person's or population's environment. The WHO (Prüss-Ustün et al, 2016, p x) defines environment, as it relates to health, as 'all the physical, chemical, and biological factors external to a person, and all the related behaviors'. Environmental health consists of preventing or controlling disease, injury and disability related to the interactions between people and their environment. Population health can be measured through statistics about levels of air pollution and emissions, noise, toxic substances, and waste against predefined safety thresholds.

Why is this important?

Definitions and models of health are important when considering and understanding health and wellbeing, and how to integrate them into impact assessments that are relevant to spatial planning. Integrating health into impact assessment at a plan, policy or proposal level can be complicated, being defined not only by an individual's view of health, but also that of society, key stakeholders, legislators, policymakers, developers and those commissioned to carry out an impact assessment that has health as an element (Cave et al, 2021; Winkler et al, 2021).

It is important that there is clarity about the process and what it entails, along with explicit regulator, professional body or legislator guidance around how these are carried out, the elements that must be considered within them and which health model is to be used as a lens. There are several forms of impact assessment that consider the population-level impact and are statutory obligations for spatial planning policies, plans and projects. Chapter 7 concentrates on these, the lens utilised and how health issues are currently incorporated into assessments across the world. It discusses the challenges in achieving the integration of health into the assessments and how these can be overcome in the short to long term.

Health and Strategic Environmental Assessment

Strategic Environmental Assessment (SEA) is applied to plans and programmes globally (Fischer, 2007; Therival, 2010). It aims to ensure that any significant environmental impacts or risks of these are identified. These include, for example, national and local spatial plans, transport plans, or waste plans. It aims to inform decision-makers and implement mitigation and monitoring once the plans or strategies have been approved or implemented. SEA is used extensively at a global level – with statutory legislation in place for it in, for example, the European Union (EU), UK and North America (European Parliament and Council of the European Union, 2001; UNECE, 2015; Government of Canada, 2019). There is a plethora of guidance and peer-reviewed literature about SEA as a process and its effectiveness (Fischer, 2007), which this chapter does not aim to replicate. It is a systematic prospective (that is, in advance of) process that has been extensively practised for 20 years and aims to inform decisions on plans and the form, content and delivery of them (UNECE, 2019).

While published papers suggest that integrating health into SEA as a process has been growing in practice, they also demonstrate that this process is still inconsistent in its focus and extent (Therival and Partido, 2013; Tajima and Fischer, 2013). Unless otherwise stated, the health determinants considered tend to be environmental health oriented and include air quality and noise, with some social and economic factors also considered. The Convention on Environmental Impact Assessment in a Transboundary Context (Espoo Convention) and the EU SEA Directive (European Parliament and Council of the European Union, 2001) state that SEA must identify the significant effects on 'human health'.

However, the term 'human health' can be defined in many ways and so can be open to interpretation; practice has evolved so that it is largely focused on the environmental model of health and quantifiable impacts and metrics (Cave et al, 2021). This is integral in defending the process and the evidence base on which it has been developed.

Guidance has recently been prepared for the United Nations Economic Committee in Europe (UNECE, 2019). This can help to strengthen health integration into SEA, as could involving public health specialists, who can assist in the identification of health impacts, how they are considered and who these will affect. This would add value to the process, as while there is guidance on the process and format of reporting, for example, in Scotland, SEA does not mandate a consideration of the different impacts across the population, which is integral to health inequalities and public health (Scottish Government, 2013).

Health and Environmental Impact Assessment

Environmental Impact Assessment (EIA) is applied to local-level projects across the world (United Nations Environment, 2018). The nature of the projects must meet criteria set out in national acts, guidance or regulations (European Parliament and Council of the European Union, 2001, 2014; Government of Canada,

2019; Brown et al, 2020), and can include, for example, transport projects, housing developments, waste management sites and energy developments (Cave et al, 2020; Winkler et al, 2020).

Similar to SEA, EIA is routinely carried out globally. Health as a consideration is also incorporated into it – with explicit reference to 'human health' in the vast majority of cases. In Europe, changes to the EU EIA Directive implemented in 2017 state that all EIAs undertaken must identify, describe and assess, in an appropriate manner, in the light of each individual case, the direct and indirect significant effects of a project on population and human health. Like an SEA, an EIA is carried out prospectively to inform decision-making, and there is a predominant focus on the environmental model of health, with some social and economic factors considered (Winkler et al, 2020). There are some examples of EIAs across the world in which requirements (or specific requests in tender briefs) consider the social determinants of health and inequalities (Benusic, 2014; RPS Group, 2015; Horizon Nuclear Power, 2018), but these have been few in number.

Global guidance has recently been published by the International Association of Impact Assessment and European Public Health Association that aims to provide a steer to those who wish, or have been commissioned, to carry out an EIA or have been given a specific remit to focus on population/human health (Cave et al, 2021). Alongside a wide range of international practitioners, the literature informed by this has identified how health has been included or practised as part of environmental assessments to date (Brown et al, 2020; Winkler et al, 2020; Cave et al, 2021).

There has also been guidance and advice published at a national level in some states about health integration. For example, the Institute of Environmental Management and Assessment (IEMA) and PHE have published England-based guidance for the incorporation of health into EIA based on the changes to the EU EIA Directive in 2017. Although these are welcome, it can add to the confusion and inconsistency in practice around health integration (Winkler et al, 2021), particularly when EIAs are scrutinised, examined and must be defended to a competent authority or regulator.

Integrated sustainability assessment and IIA

Health is routinely integrated into the SEA/EIA process (Cave et al, 2021) if a standalone HIA has not been commissioned. Where multiple, separate assessments are required by law, local policy context and practice, for example, HIA, social impact assessment (Vanclay, 2003) or indigenous language or cultural impact assessments (Croal et al, 2012), these are often woven together into a joint impact assessment framework, which has a single scope, interconnected evidence-gathering processes and evidence base. The aim is to have shared outcomes, for example, one comprehensive report with a set of monitoring data. These can be described as integrated sustainability assessment (ISA) or IIA for a plan or policy, and/or environmental and social impact assessment (ESIA) or environmental, social and health impact assessment (ESHIA) for a project.

As a multidisciplinary approach and process, this makes sense to maximise resources. However, if this approach is followed, then the health and/or wellbeing and inequalities components must be made explicit within the scoping stages (along with the other integrated elements to be considered, such as social, environmental or cultural impacts). A challenge with this type of process is the potential for confusion, not only in its content (which can be avoided and clarified through strong scope, aims and objectives), but also in the terminology used to describe these processes. Omission of these early elements is hugely important, as these component parts of the process influence the nature and content of the impact assessment and the way that it is carried out. If public health or health-focused planning officers miss this window, then the 'window of opportunity' to influence the impact assessment can be lost.

Mental wellbeing impact assessment

Mental wellbeing impact assessment (MWIA) is a related tool to HIA and follows a similar systematic, flexible and evidenced-based approach to assessing, promoting and measuring the impact of a policy, proposal or plan on mental wellbeing (Cooke et al, 2011). It can be beneficial to policy- and decision-makers in the practical implementation and integration of mental wellbeing, and can have a major role in reviewing and redesigning services or change in organisations (Health Knowledge, 2021; PHW, 2021b).

Like other assessments, MWIA provides a structured framework for involving stakeholders to identify specific impacts on mental wellbeing of developments, programmes, services, policies and organisations. It can provide evidence-based recommendations to maximise any identified positive impacts and minimise or mitigate potential negative impacts. The process is particularly focused on four key protective factors for mental wellbeing:

- enhancing a sense of control;
- building emotional resilience and community assets, such as social networks and places to participate and engage with others;
- promoting participation and inclusion, such as a sense of community and place; and
- wider socio-economic factors with an impact on mental wellbeing, such as levels of income, employment, environment, housing and transport.

Evidence demonstrates that these factors can all promote or inhibit mental wellbeing and health equalities. It explicitly considers the latter by highlighting the populations whose mental health and wellbeing will be particularly positively or negatively affected by the plan or development proposal, and allows for the mitigation of any negative impact. There is clear guidance, criteria and tools available to follow (Cooke et al, 2011).

While MWIA is not a statutory process anywhere in the world, it can be an additional option for policy, project and plan makers where the psychological and mental wellbeing impact of proposals is identified as significant. It may not seem an immediately obvious process for spatial planners (or public health professionals) to undertake, but it can be a valuable tool when appropriate, depending on the context, situation and planning proposal. MWIA can be applied to any development or service where there is an opportunity to promote positive, or need to mitigate negative, mental wellbeing impacts (Table 6.1).

Table 6.1: Relating impact assessments to the models of health

Model	Impact assessment typology			
	HIA	SEA	EIA	MWIA
Medical	√			√
Holistic	√ (dependent on tender brief, scope and context)	√ (dependent on tender brief, scope and context)	√ (dependent on tender brief, scope and context)	√
Wellness	√			√
Environmental	√	√	√	

MWIA has been applied to environmental projects, green space developments, libraries and education, workplaces, housing and regeneration plans and projects, health and social care services, and community and third sector projects and services (Cooke and Stansfield, 2009).

Maximise planning and health value in impact assessments

All the impact assessments discussed earlier have scope for a consideration of health, wellbeing and vulnerable groups at the population level to a greater or lesser extent. This is highly dependent on the model of health that they utilise. However, there are opportunities to shape the perspective on health taken during the impact assessment process itself (whichever perspective or sector you come from) through the discussions about scoping and any inclusion/exclusion criteria as part of the process.

There is a requirement for a scoping stage to be completed for all of these assessments. In the amended EU EIA Directive, population and health are included in the formal scoping process. HIA and health can be integrated into this stage, and a distinct HIA scoping exercise can be carried out to inform the scoping statement or opinion, which provides an important opportunity to identify and include key public health and health services stakeholders other than the statutory consultees. This is the most effective point to fully integrate health or a standalone HIA, as the scope is established and the methods and the necessary outputs are agreed. Once agreed, the scope must be delivered and will provide clear criteria for the appraisal of evidence. The deliverable may be 'a distinct, standalone HIA (driven by local or sector specific policy), and/or a population and health chapter in a report. Ultimately, the principles, process and outputs are the same, but the reporting and document structure that changes' (A. Buroni, personal correspondence). Any standalone HIA report can be entered as a technical appendix, and the evidence obtained from it can be included in any more streamlined population and health chapter of the EIA or SEA.

Challenge in defining health in planning

The aim of the planning system is the allocation of land for transport planning and travel links, and for economic development, housing and other development types. However, in doing so, it can also lead to better or poorer health and wellbeing. Health is routinely considered as part of spatial planning-related impact assessments across the world, and there is legislation in place to ensure this, for example: the Japan Environmental Impact Assessment Act 1997; the Canada Environmental Assessment Act 2012 and Impact Assessment Act 2019; the 2001 and 2014 Directives of the European Parliament; and the Public Health (Wales) Act 2017.

In the context of public health-focused spatial planning that analyses plans using a population health-level lens of health protection, health promotion and healthcare services, there needs to be a move away from the environmental model of health that is routinely utilised to the holistic or wellness models of health and equity. This poses several challenges, including terminology, interpretation, legislation, practical guidance, knowledge, understanding and skills, rigour and defensibility, and economics. However, it can be achieved and integrated in this way, as demonstrated by several ISAs, EIAs and SEAs carried out internationally (Tajima and Fischer, 2013; Cave et al, 2021; Winkler et al, 2020, 2021; Welsh Government, 2021b).

Health is integral to everyone and their communities (WHO, 1986). A person's experience of being healthy or not can shape their own and their community's views of life. Similarly, health and wellbeing are integral to spatial planning sectors, the public health system and, more importantly, the communities that are subject to plans, policies and development projects and their processes. For the lens to become more public health inclusive, there are key issues and challenges that need to be worked through.

There are challenges to health integration, including: the definition of health followed and the understanding of this by a wide range of actors, such as assessors, commissioners, competent authorities or regulators, and developers; the economic development drivers that may take precedence; legal obligations; the extent and timing of involvement by health and public health stakeholders; and the lack of public health capacity to input into the assessment process or review it (Cave et al, 2020, 2021; Winkler et al, 2021).

The definitions of health are not defined in regulations and are therefore open to interpretation. Health and wellbeing also include tangible and intangible determinants of health, and consist of individuals' and communities' perceptions and priorities, which can be widely differing. These can be complicated further at an individual level by a person's lived experience and values. This can be overcome by clear guidance at an international or national level that has explicit significance criteria and defines what health means and which model of health it refers to.

Public health is an 'art and a science', which needs to be critically unpicked and agreed. The guidance needs to not only involve consultation with regulators, legislators and key stakeholders, such as spatial planners, environmental and national public health institutes and local communities, but also actively engage them from the start of the process.

Challenge of health sector consultation

There is the challenge of *who exactly* you consult in the health sector. There are public health institutes at a national (and regional) level in many nation states, but in others, there are health protection agencies, health boards and health agencies, health services delivery bodies with estates management responsibilities, hospital trusts, and so on. These often then have local teams, which adds confusion, and it can be hard for those carrying out assessments to be able to engage with the right people. Again, clear legislator, professional organisation and regulator-approved guidance can help, as well as the support of a dedicated public health and spatial planning team, for example, a single point of contact, as in Wales via the WHIASU.

Statutory consultees are often listed and defined in guidance, and these need to include the government-recognised national public health institute or public health agency, as well as health services or estates. Some nations have guidance for different types of assessments, for example, in Wales (Cave et al, 2021), but in the main, there is an absence of guidance, leading to inconsistent practice. In terms of health integration and standalone HIAs that can be incorporated into the wider process, some guidance exists that aims to support spatial planners and public health officers to maximise any opportunities that may exist to enable healthy planning and development as part of the plan-making and development process.

Role of experts

Consultants who carry out assessments tend to focus on their particular area of expertise, such as toxicology, noise or air quality, as part of a multidisciplinary team in the private sector. By their nature, SEAs and EIAs are complex due to the range of topics to be assessed; therefore, multidisciplinary and specialist teams are essential. However, this means that they can be expensive to carry out and defend in front of planning inspectors or regulators. Environmental assessments are often commissioned by developers, who aim to maximise their profits, but this can lead to conflict, as any processes and outputs that are not required by law, for example, HIAs that are social determinant and equity focused, may be dispensed with due to economics and legal obligations.

Specialist skills and knowledge are the key to a robust and high-quality assessment, along with the ability to defend it to commissioners and regulators, for example, at a public inquiry.

This is important, and a registered public health specialist will be able to perform this function within the boundaries of the guidance and legislation.

Driving force for considering health in assessments

Policymakers are frequently driven to focus on the potential economic benefits of plans and projects in terms of gross domestic product (GDP), as well as any societal and associated employment opportunities, such as housing growth. The latter do have benefits to health and wellbeing, but any wider implications of a project or plan should also be considered.

Such frameworks as the UN SDGs could provide another method of driving a wider consideration of the impacts of a project or plan for a range of sectors, as these SDGs include health, environment, equity and economy (Buss et al, 2019; Rogerson et al, 2020). Planners who commission, monitor and approve plans and projects need to consult with their local or national public health stakeholders to ensure that while the benefits of plans and developments are maximised and highlighted, any mitigation of detrimental health inequalities are similarly considered and implemented, ensuring that any pre-agreed measures to improve local infrastructure, such as local healthcare services or roads, are carried out in a timely way and to the levels agreed as part of planning permissions or approvals.

One way of mitigating negative impacts and maximising benefits would be by building in the health enablers from the start of a developmental or plan lifecycle, not at the end as an afterthought. This is where such approaches as HiAP and supportive processes like HIA are important. Examples include building cycle lanes from the start of housing development construction or building in and landscaping green space in the first phase so that the residents who live in these developments gain health benefits from the outset, not several years after they have lived in it and have become used to using a car to shop or access local facilities, including green or blue space. The former approach builds in health and wellness, while the latter can lead to the creation of obesogenic environments and behaviour, for example, through the lack of opportunity to take active travel and physical activity, leading to reliance on a car and, in turn, possibly poor health outcomes (Johnson and Green, 2021).

Integrating health in assessments

In relation to health integration and linked to the challenges noted in Chapter 5, there is the need for more support, training and capacity building for both planners and public health specialists (Harris et al, 2014). As previously highlighted, the lack of public health capacity to engage with HIA and health in other impact assessment processes, such as EIA and SEA, is a challenge (Winkler et al, 2020). Public health officers and health assessors also need to recognise and better understand core requirements in relation to accountability and the need to be able to robustly defend any health element of an assessment, the evidence used, the process followed and the findings. Wider health, wellbeing and equity-focused assessments need to be mindful of this from the outset, alongside recognising the overlap with other technical disciplines that are protective of the environment and health (Green et al, 2021a).

The integration of health or HIA into regulatory assessments, such as SEA and EIA processes, requires a pragmatic approach and clear objectives and scope (Cave et al, 2017; Brown et al, 2020; Pyper et al, 2021). It also requires the ability to connect and coordinate with wider technical disciplines, such as toxicology or air quality, and a clear understanding that the work will need to be robustly defended in particular forums.

Environmental-related assessments need to evolve in order to become much more focused on public health, wider determinants and inequalities. In the absence of this, assessors should do the best that they can while also trying to influence the content of guidance and legislation (should they so wish) to change the emphasis from one of a model of risk and environmental health, to one that is more holistic and wellness driven.

It must also be recognised that different nation states are at different points in the evolution and integration of health, wellbeing and equity in spatial planning and development implementation (Rogerson et al, 2020). In some nations in the world, for example, the UK, Canada, Thailand, parts of Europe and other economically developed and sustainable development-aware countries, public health and planning practitioners are pushing for a shift in the way health is considered in spatial planning, and this is gaining traction.

However, it must be noted that there are many countries that are simply pushing for basic environmental and biophysical health risks to be considered as part of policies, plans and projects. This means that for public health and environmental protection officers in these countries, the inclusion of health per se is important, rather than the definition and model – and the wellness model of promoting health and wellbeing is an ambition, rather than a reality. It is even more important that the policy and practice context be considered when integrating health into plans and development proposals.

Opportunities for health in integrated assessments

Taking a collaborative approach and a holistic view of health and wellbeing can 'add value':

- strengthening plans and projects so that they are appropriate for the community;
- considering the social determinants of health, which includes environmental and economic impacts;
- promoting due diligence by instigating mitigation and monitoring processes;
- utilising such tools as HIA to identify both positive and negative impacts of plans of projects; and
- promoting engagement, discussions and access to evidence in consultation stages, including as regards health intelligence data from key stakeholders like public health and healthcare services and systems, as early engagement with local or national public health stakeholders can unlock a variety of data and evidence, and provide access to a range of perspectives, to mitigate detrimental health and equalities issues at the start of the development process.

There are opportunities for health integration to take place. Legislation can often allow for health input into the development of plans and projects (European Parliament and Council of the European Union, 2014; UNECE, 2019; Brown et al, 2020; Cave et al, 2021). This can be achieved in small steps. As an example, in Wales, the Public Health (Wales) Act 2017 will enable more HIAs to be carried out for SEAs of development plans, and 'Planning Policy Wales' (Welsh Government, 2021a) has a requirement for wider health to be considered as part of development planning, with HIAs either to be carried out as a standalone process or to be integrated into the SEA. Similarly, the third edition of the 'Local Development Plan Manual' (Welsh Government, 2020) outlines the use of HIA as a valuable tool. Both specify national HIA guidance that must be followed, which has an emphasis on the social determinants of health and wellbeing.

There is available support, resources, guides and training to enable a better understanding and promote capacity building for health integration or a consideration of health and wellbeing into other impact assessments. National public health institutes (PHE, Public Health Wales and Public Health Scotland in the UK, and the Institute of Public Health in Ireland) publish guides and host training events on health integration into planning or HIA as a standalone process, as do public health associations (European Public Health Association). Practitioner bodies, such as the International Association for Impact Assessment (IAIA), IEMA and Society of Practitioners of Health Impact Assessment (SOPHIA), also provide guidance, training and resources, as do organisations such as WHO regional offices and collaborating centres (for example, the Centres on Environmental Health Impact Assessment, Health in Impact Assessment and Investment for Health and Wellbeing), and academic institutions (for example, the Centre for Health Equity Training Research and Evaluation [CHETRE] in Australia). It has also been highlighted that health practitioners and assessors can learn from the knowledge and practice of other impact assessments (Morgan, 2011; Cave et al, 2021).

Concluding statement

This chapter has focused on integrating health into the different types of other impact assessments, including those for which there is a regulatory requirement for spatial plans and projects, and it notes some of the challenges in doing this. The successful integration of health or HIA as a process into EIA and SEA can be enabled by some small steps: overcoming misconceptions from all sides of the systems by understanding others' perspectives and terminology; knowing the actual detail of the policy and regulatory assessment requirements, and what the sectors or communities are trying to achieve; outlining clearly what is being sought; and recognising that the underlying aim of HIA is the same as SEA or EIA, and that all the processes outlined in this chapter have the same intention at their core – to inform and refine a policy, plan or proposal, and to assist and influence decision-making.

Insider story 6.1: Using the HIA to embed health into the LDP in Cardiff, Wales

Stuart Williams, Cardiff Council's Group Leader (Policy), shares his experience of applying an HIA to the creation of Cardiff's LDP. Cardiff is the capital city of Wales, with a population of just under 367,000 people, and it plays an important role within the region in providing housing and jobs. Welsh government guidance requires the council to prepare and regularly update an LDP for the area, which sets out future growth in terms of homes and jobs, important environmental areas for protection, and a range of policies to assess development proposals against.

The council began work on the LDP in 2011, and early in the evidence-gathering process, health was identified as a key issue that the plan needed to address. Evidence showed that Cardiff has a relatively prosperous north and a southern arc of deprivation, with a 20-year gap in life expectancy between the two areas. Allied to this, it also found that 51 per cent of the population were classified as overweight or obese.

Given this, it was important to ensure that health issues were embedded in the plan preparation process, and in conjunction with the local health board, the council determined that HIA would be the most appropriate tool to use because:

- it is a relatively straightforward and systematic process, allowing changes to be suggested for each individual policy in the LDP;
- it allows an iterative process to be followed, with HIA undertaken at key stages in LDP preparation;
- it enables an audit trail of how health issues have been addressed for the LDP examination;
- it results in improved policies/plans, which are more effective as a result; and
- training and advice are available on undertaking HIA with WHIASU.

It was determined that the most appropriate methodology to use was the template set out in the WHIASU's (2012) *Health Impact Assessment: A Practical Guide*, which assesses the effects of policies against a range of health issues, including healthy lifestyles, housing quality, access to work, accessibility, food access, climate change, crime reduction and community safety, air quality and neighbourhood amenity, social cohesion and social capital, public services, and resource minimisation.

In order to ensure a robust assessment, the HIA was undertaken by a group with representatives from Cardiff and the Vale Health Board, the WHIASU and various departments within Cardiff Council, including planning, transport, environment and sustainability. Each LDP policy was assessed in terms of positive and negative impacts, and suggested mitigating actions were documented, together with how the council would respond to these actions. A report setting out the findings and recommendations of the HIA was prepared at the two key stages in the LDP preparation process. The HIA process for the LDP identified the following issues to address:

- provide sustainable transport infrastructure, accessible services and community facilities up front so that they are available for future residents to use from the outset;
- provide good-quality, accessible open space;
- provide infrastructure to support walking and cycling, including segregated cycle routes;
- ensure new homes are energy efficient;
- provide a range of types of new housing;
- reuse topsoil;
- provide community growing space and allotments;

- provide measures to ensure community safety; and
- mitigate potential air, noise and light pollution.

These issues were considered when drafting the policies to include in the LDP. In order to focus on the issue and ensure health is fully taken into account in new development proposals, it was considered necessary to depart from established practice and include two specific LDP policies relating to heath. These policies prioritise reducing health inequalities and encouraging healthy lifestyles through supporting developments that provide for active travel and accessible and useable green spaces, including allotments. They also require priority to be given in new developments for providing sites for new accessible health facilities. The LDP was adopted in 2016, and since then, supplementary planning guidance on planning for health and wellbeing has been produced to complement the health policies in the adopted LDP and provide more detailed information to developers on potential health impacts and the ways these can be mitigated in new developments.

What is the overall observable lesson?

It was clear that the benefits to the council in adding value to the LDP preparation process and final document outweighed the limitations:

- It is important to recognise that undertaking the HIA is a learning process and the team will develop knowledge over time, and that the process is flexible, so you can tailor it to suit your requirements.
- HIA is a positive approach – it seeks to look not only at the negatives, but also at the positives – and is a vehicle for promoting cross-department and cross-sector working, and for incorporating different viewpoints and ideas into policy development.
- Importantly, HIA can help reduce the potential negative impacts on health by thinking about the way policies are written and considering the short- and long-term impacts, along with obvious and less obvious impacts.

In terms of limitations, it is important that staff undertaking the process have training so that they fully understand the process, and in this respect, examples of HIA successfully undertaken elsewhere are useful. Allied to this, it is also beneficial when undertaking a self-assessment to have people in the assessment team with knowledge of health issues. It is important to manage expectations, as not all recommendations can be taken on board because the LDP needs to be prepared in accordance with Welsh government guidance and certain recommendations may not be in tune with this guidance or may be undeliverable or unviable.

The process for undertaking the HIA and the way in which the council translated the recommendations into the LDP policies were subject to scrutiny by the planning inspectors appointed to undertake the examination of the LDP. They concluded that the approach taken by the council was sound and no significant changes to the health policies were recommended by the inspectors.

Further information

The 2016 Cardiff LDP is available at: www.cardiffldp.co.uk/adopted-local-development-plan

The Cardiff 'Planning for health and wellbeing: supplementary planning guidance' is available at: www.cardiff.gov.uk/ENG/resident/Planning/Planning-Policy/Supplementary-Planning-Guidance/Documents/Planning%20for%20Health%20and%20Wellbeing%20SPG.pdf

Insider story 6.2: Integrating health, wellbeing and inequalities in 'Future Wales'

Gemma Christian, Planning Manager in the Planning Directorate of the Welsh government, shares her insight into the process of integrating health into Wales' national plan. 'Future Wales' has set the direction for development in Wales for the next 20 years. It is a development plan with a strategy for addressing key national priorities through the planning system, including: sustaining and developing a vibrant economy; achieving decarbonisation and climate resilience; developing strong ecosystems; and improving the health and wellbeing of communities. 'Future Wales' takes an HiAP approach, which reflects the diverse impact that planning has on health, wellbeing and inequality.

The impact assessment of 'Future Wales' is a Welsh government project, a national-scale assessment fundamentally shaped by the goals and ways of working of the Well-being of Future Generations Act. The preparation of 'Future Wales' has been underpinned by the integrated sustainability appraisal (ISA). This incorporates the sustainability appraisal, SEA, equalities, children's rights, economic development, health, rural-proofing, climate change and Welsh language impact assessments. The different assessments were required by a mix of legislation and national policy to ensure 'Future Wales' is sustainable. They also ensured transparency at each stage of plan development, setting out the options and choices that were made, and helped to inform engagement and involvement with the plan.

The processes of undertaking impact assessments on development plans are well established, and this knowledge and experience helped to shape the approach to assessing 'Future Wales'. It was at the very early screening stage that the clear overlaps and potential opportunities and benefits to integrating the different assessments were explored.

The decision to integrate an HIA, though not required by legislation, acknowledged the recognition of the important links between planning and health, wellbeing and inequalities, and the wider determinants of health. Once the scope of the project was set, a team was established to undertake the assessments, formed of consultants and members of the

'Future Wales' team, who worked together to co-produce the assessment. This ensured that the assessment was undertaken collaboratively and iteratively throughout the development of the plan, guaranteeing that the outcomes of the assessment shaped and improved the plan.

The SEA regulations approach was the starting point to structure the assessment process, and was adapted using the Well-being of Future Generations Act and requirements of the various impact assessments to produce an ISA. This approach provides a consistent methodology across the different assessments. The ISA framework was shaped by evidence, engagement and consultation, and was reviewed at each stage of the plan as it developed. It contained 17 objectives, with decision-aiding questions that helped to structure the consideration of impacts. This resulted in recommendations for improving the plan. This iterative process flagged up potential impacts early on, enabling the policies and proposals to address these impacts and maximise opportunities for health, wellbeing and inequality.

The opportunity to reduce duplication will continue through a joint monitoring framework for the plan and the assessment work. This will feed into future reviews of the plan to provide a robust evidence base and for the identification of trends and impacts.

This integrated approach has ensured that the variety of impacts, including on health, wellbeing and inequality, have been discussed and considered in a collaborative manner. It helped to: share knowledge and recognise links between different areas; ensure a consistent approach to and level of detail for each of the different assessments; and demonstrate the evolution of 'Future Wales', such as why decisions were made, what options were considered and the opportunities to maximise positive benefits and avoid or minimise negative impact. This meant that the impacts were recognised at the earliest stage and led to the production of a robust assessment that has ensured 'Future Wales' is as sustainable as possible.

What is the overall observable lesson?

The integrated approach to assessing the plan has resulted in a holistic and robust assessment, which recognises the role of planning in delivering benefits and avoiding or minimising negative impacts. Involvement and engagement have been key, and this has included assessment-specific workshops, webinars, accessible versions of documents, conferences and formal consultation. Bringing different stakeholders together in a collaborative and iterative way to discuss issues and impacts enables the range of determinants of health, wellbeing and inequality to be looked at alongside social, economic, cultural and environmental issues, and to be considered throughout all aspects of the plan.

Ensuring this work starts early and planning the project well will help to create a robust assessment that clearly shapes a plan or policy, testing options and exploring opportunities at the earliest stage. It is also important to put in place systems to keep the evidence under review. There are opportunities to streamline processes, such as monitoring, data collection and consultation, throughout the different stages of plan development.

Further information

'Future Wales: the national plan 2040' is available at: https://gov.wales/future-wales-national-plan-2040

PART III

Actions to improve practice

> New requirements, processes, structures and new
> languages will require local authority planners and
> public health professionals to learn how things work
> in practice. This presents new opportunities.
>
> Chang and Ross (2012, p 307)

Tangible progress is being made on planning for health as practitioners utilise the planning powers and levers available to them within the legislative and policy parameters set out by governments to deliver local public health outcomes. The planning system provides a number of entry points and opportunities to build in health and wellbeing, from policy development and plan making (upstream), to the decisions made on urban development projects and the mechanisms used to secure and finance healthy developments (downstream). Examples of innovative and good practices are constantly emerging, and some of these are highlighted and widely communicated to practitioners to learn key lessons.

While it is important to appreciate that we are not starting from square one, there is a recognition that the state of practice is not static or sequential, but rather multifaceted, multidimensional and evolutionary. In practice, the art and science of planning for health relies on the commitment of individuals and of professions in statutory and non-statutory settings, and is premised on the evolution of systems and rules.

As systems and rules are changed, replaced, improved, deregulated or even removed, the state of practice will transform. Similarly, as individuals move on from jobs, change teams or departments, or take on new responsibilities, the state of practice will also transform as a result. Improving public health spatial planning in practice cannot rely on personal relationships alone. That is why it is important to identify how the required competencies should be reflected in the education of future generations of professionals, as well as in the professional development of those currently in practice.

This part of the book recognises that an understanding of the state of current practice can help practitioners:

- acknowledge and learn from the progress that has been made across the end-to-end stages of the planning system and processes;
- consider where past mistakes have been made to enable improvements, and to identify areas to focus on in the future that make the greatest impact; and
- follow up on learning from examples and adapt them to their day-to-day practice.

It also enables readers to:

- understand how best to integrate health and wellbeing in policy development at national and local levels (see Chapter 7);
- understand how health and wellbeing considerations can best be integrated in urban development decision-making processes (see Chapter 8); and
- understand what skills are needed to begin to establish a competency framework to become an effective public health spatial planning practitioner (see Chapter 9).

Part III key takeaways

- Integrating health and wellbeing considerations during the development of spatial plans and policies is a prerequisite for making healthy and sound local planning decisions.
- Adopting the eight-stage process for healthy planning policy development can help create strong policies that can command authority and consensus among stakeholders.

- Considering public health considerations in planning decisions should go beyond just policy compliance and take a wider public interest perspective.
- Involving public health professionals in the process is integral to ensuring that spatial plans, policies and decisions reflect local health and wellbeing needs.
- Improving the capacity and capability of current and future practitioners through educational and professional development systems is critical to sustaining a pipeline of competent professionals.

7

Health and wellbeing in planning policy

> We can, if we choose, legislate, subsidize, and plan
> for health promotion and disease prevention ... We
> must have the master plans, the building codes, the
> tax policies, the knowledge, and the leadership to
> enact this kind of solution.
>
> Dannenberg et al (2011, pp xvii–xviii)

The planning system operates on the primacy of legislative and
policy frameworks as the basis for action. This hierarchical nature
of spatial planning is a hallmark of the system and dictates how
regional/local authorities and stakeholders are able and required
to embed health and wellbeing into strategies, plans and policies.

There are different models to explain the policy development
process and function (Nutbeam, 2020), and many health-related
planning policies are a combination of these models or start with
one but evolve into another:

- *Knowledge-driven*: informed by new or changing evidence
  about particular interventions or lessons from practice.
- *Problem-solving*: informed by a need to take remedial action
  to address policy or practical challenges, or to meet targets
  and legislative requirements.
- *Interactive*: informed by pressure, lobbying and changing
  discourse from stakeholders and special interest groups.
- *Political*: driven by a particular political ideology and
  predetermined position.

- *Tactical*: informed by changing trends and patterns, but not necessarily yet supported by evidence.

This chapter makes the case for the integration of health and wellbeing issues into the policy framework, how to do this and the types of policies needed that are robust and defensible, and that can be tailored to meet local spatial and public health priorities, such as those set out in public health strategies. Most importantly, this chapter provides policymakers and practitioners with the necessary know-how to translate evidence and knowledge into policy and technical requirements. It highlights:

- 'gateways' or opportunities for public health involvement in planning policy development at various administrative and spatial levels; and
- processes and principles for robust, deliverable policy requirements on health.

Who is involved in developing policy?

Policy development does not operate in a vacuum and is often a process and result of interaction and relationships between multiple actors:

- The national department: responsible for formulating policy directions, adjudicating the process and reporting to national politicians.
- The planning authority: responsible for policy development and decision-making, and is the gatekeeper and foundational administrative unit for planning and public health responsibilities and functions.
- Technical consultees: responsible for specialist expertise and input as either statutory or non-statutory parties in the planning process.
- Third-party interests: a range of stakeholders with interests, including non-governmental organisations, private sector investors and developers, such as those identified in Figure 3.1.

- Communities: members of the general public, including community groupings in the locality, with an interest in and/ or who will be impacted by policy.

Setting health within different levels of the spatial planning hierarchy

Each level of the planning system hierarchy provides different scope and parameters for public health issues to be integrated. Each level has a different implementer or responsible authority, which adds a dimension of complexity across a whole country. The hierarchy stages and the strength of the policies they develop will vary in different countries according to geopolitical arrangements. They will also differ according to whether power and policy responsibilities are concentrated at the top or devolved geographically to lower-tier authorities. If the former, the specificity and prescription of policy needed will be greater at the national level, while the latter arrangement will see this level of specificity and prescription lighter at national but stronger at the lower, devolved tiers of policy development.

Each level provides a gateway for public health involvement and opportunity for health and wellbeing issues to be integrated. This hierarchy of gateways consists of:

1. national-level policy and guidance;
2. strategic-level policy and guidance;
3. local-level policy and guidance; and
4. neighbourhood and site-level policy and guidance.

National-level policy and guidance

National planning strategies, policies or directives will set out the government's planning policies for the country and how they should be applied, and will provide a framework within which lower tiers of planning strategies or policies should be followed and created. These are often articulated in the form of legislation and policy documents. For example, in England, the Planning and Compulsory Purchase Act 2004 (as amended by subsequent legislation) gives effect to the status of the National Planning Policy Framework (NPPF) in the planning hierarchy. The responsible authority at this level is mainly the national or federal department accountable for spatial planning policy. Politicians and policymakers need to recognise the trickle-down effect of policies where weak or non-existent intentions regarding promoting health and wellbeing and reducing inequalities can undermine efforts at the lower-tier policy and guidance levels. However, in decentralised arrangements, where there are more devolved powers and responsibilities for legislative policymaking, national-level policy and guidance may not play as a great a role as they do in more centralised systems.

The benefits of creating a health planning policy requirement at this level are to ensure:

- a clarity of intent, signalling a policy direction on health and wellbeing to those decision-makers in lower tiers, while retaining flexibility to reflect varying circumstances of larger geographies, populations and their health needs; and
- permission, signalling the parameters of mandatory and discretionary public health consideration, which often form the basis of 'policy hooks' on which local planning for health policies and decisions are made.

Healthy places in Wales planning policy

'Planning Policy Wales', edition 11 (Welsh Government, 2021a) translates wider Welsh government objectives and strategies into planning policy, and guides decisions for local planning authorities. Under 'Promoting healthier places', the Welsh government states that planning 'should identify proactive and preventative measures to reduce health inequalities. This will include enabling opportunities for outdoor activity and recreation, reducing exposure of populations to air and noise pollution, promoting active travel options and seeking environmental and physical improvements, particularly in the built environment' (Welsh Government, 2021a).

Strategic-level policy and guidance

Below the national level, there will be strategic planning authorities at the large geographical units of regions, sub-regions or larger-than-local policies. Often, there will be a requirement for this level of policy development to be in compliance, take into account or be in general conformity with national-level policy and guidance. In addition, there will be a requirement to avoid repeating national policy verbatim, so such policies and guidance will often adapt national policy to ensure they include sufficient details of strategic importance to the locality.

The benefits of creating a health planning policy requirement at this level are to ensure:

- consensus of importance, where strategic authorities agree on the strategic significance of health and wellbeing issues across a large geographic locality;
- cooperation, where strategic authorities can cooperate constructively, actively and on an ongoing basis to maximise the effectiveness of strategic health policies, particularly relating to health and social care infrastructure investments; and
- consistency of strategy, where strategic policies or even the evidence base can provide a level of consistency to underpin a single policy approach for lower-tier authorities to implement.

Strategic London policy for promoting healthy food access

The mayor of London has planning powers across Greater London, while the 33 individual lower-tier boroughs also have planning powers. The mayor's 'Spatial development strategy' was adopted in March 2021 and introduces Policy E9C, which requires boroughs to manage over-concentrations of hot-food takeaway uses in town centres and prohibits such uses within a 400-metre walking distance of primary and secondary schools on the grounds of helping to reduce childhood obesity. The government inspector determined the matter to be of strategic importance to London, not just a detailed matter for individual boroughs.

Local-level policy and guidance

Local municipal governments are at the vanguard of setting detailed policy requirements, developing technical guidance and implementing these on programmes and projects. This level forms the primary local planning framework. In the UK, it is often referred to as the 'plan-led' system, where planning law dictates planning decisions to be made in accordance with the adopted local plan, unless there are other material considerations (for more on material considerations, see Chapter 8).

The local policy framework is required to be compliant with the parameters set out in higher-level policies and guidance (national and strategic). This compliance provides both challenges (for example, stifling local innovation where higher-level policies are silent on key health matters) and opportunities (for example, meeting minimum quality standards on housing space and green infrastructure). Challenges and opportunities are mostly influenced by the degree of political and professional commitment, as well as resources, of the local authority to develop meaningful and deliverable planning for health policies and guidance. However, integrating health into local plans is key (NHS England, 2019) and often the basis from which planning for health actions are taken.

Health and wellbeing policy in the Harlow local plan

Harlow Council in Essex, England, adopted its statutory plan in December 2020. Policy L4 on health and wellbeing states:

The Council will seek to deliver development and growth which has a positive impact on the health and wellbeing of residents, and address issues of health deprivation and health inequality in the district in accordance with the objectives of the Harlow Health and Wellbeing Strategy and in response to the various Evidence Base sources. When promoting development, applicants should consider the impact on the health and wellbeing of new and existing residents.

For the first time, a review undertaken by the TCPA in England and Wales provides a snapshot of health-relevant requirements in statutory local plans, including health references for sustainable transport, open space provision, design and the use of Health Impact Assessment (for England, see Table 7.1; for Wales, see Table 7.2). The TCPA's policy review highlights that the local planning system is embedding health considerations and that there are clear policy hooks for planning and health. Other reviews on fast-food outlet policies (Keeble et al, 2019) and older people's housing needs (Lichfields, 2018a) provide further evidence of the evolution in planning policy and practice towards health-relevant topics.

Technical guidance is supplementary and subordinate to policies but plays an important role in setting out many of the detailed requirements and processes not appropriate to a long-winded policy or policy document. Although they are resource intensive, guidance documents often do not undergo the same rigorous public policy development process (which can often take years) and are therefore an attractive tool for efficiently introducing health issues into the planning system. For example, local authorities have created guidance on a wide range of planning topics, including healthy places, sustainable housing design, HIAs and healthier food provision in hot-food takeaways, among others.

Planning for health and wellbeing guidance for Cardiff

Cardiff City in Wales developed supplementary planning guidance in November 2017 in support of its statutory planning policies. It aims to provide supporting information and guidance for planners, developers and investors, to help achieve the council's vision of addressing health inequalities, and to ensure that planning decisions contribute to achieving the goals of the Well-being of Future Generations (Wales) Act 2015.

The benefits of creating a health planning policy requirement at this level are to ensure:

Table 7.1: Review of policy in local plans in England

	Joint Health and Wellbeing Strategy in planning — Does the local plan reference the Joint Health and Wellbeing Strategy?		Health needs assessment in planning — Does the local plan take into account the local health needs set out in the Joint Strategic Needs Assessment		Promoting sustainable transport — Does the local plan promote opportunities for active travel?			Requiring good design — Does the local plan require good design in development?			Providing open space, play and recreation opportunities — Does the local plan provide opportunities for open space, play and recreation?			Healthcare infrastructure provision — Does the local plan set out provision for healthcare infrastructure?			Using HIA — Does the local plan require an HIA when a planning application is submitted?		Monitoring indicators and health (HIA) — Are there indicators that can help to monitor health impacts and benefits?	
Percentage of the total plan sample (322 Local Plans)																				
England	23	77	27	73	74	25	1	55	45	0	91	9	0	99	1	0	30	70	87	13
London	58	42	64	36	85	15	0	64	36	0	91	9	0	100	0	0	55	45	97	3
South East	9	91	8	92	58	41	1	39	59	2	89	11	0	98	2	0	14	86	86	14
South West	8	92	22	78	70	27	3	59	38	3	89	8	3	100	0	0	46	54	81	19
East	23	77	23	77	63	35	2	49	51	0	83	17	0	100	0	0	39	61	92	8
West Midlands	20	80	20	80	83	17	0	67	33	0	100	0	0	100	0	0	17	83	80	20
East Midlands	30	70	46	54	66	34	0	68	32	0	96	5	0	100	0	0	25	75	83	17
Yorkshire and the Humber	33	67	38	62	76	24	0	67	33	0	100	0	0	95	5	0	19	81	95	5
North East	8	92	25	75	75	25	0	67	33	0	75	25	0	92	8	0	25	75	75	25
North West	22	78	22	78	89	11	0	40	60	0	92	8	0	100	0	0	30	70	89	11

Yes – or (as relevant) yes, and with reference to health and wellbeing

Yes, but with no reference to health and wellbeing

No

Source: TCPA (2019). For a larger version of this table, please see: https://tcpa.org.uk/wp-content/uploads/2021/11/TCPA_5-Years-of-Health.pdf

Table 7.2: Review of policy in LDPs in Wales

Health strategy in planning	Promoting sustainable transport	Requiring good design	Providing sport and recreation opportunities	Providing green spaces	Health infrastructure provision	Using HIA	Monitoring and review
Does the LDP reference the health strategy?	Does the LDP promote opportunities for active travel?	Does the LDP require good design in development?	Does the LDP make provision for recreational opportunities?	Does the LDP make provision for green infrastructure?	Does the LDP set out provision of healthcare infrastructure?	LDP require an HIA when a planning application is submitted?	Are there indicators that can help to monitor health impacts and benefits?
77	82	45	68	82	86	5	91
23	18	55	32	18	14	95	9
0	0	0	0	0	14		

Percentage of the total plan sample (22 Local Development Plans)

Yes – or (as relevant) yes, and with reference to health and wellbeing

Yes, but with no reference to health and wellbeing

No

Source: TCPA (2019)

- that local health matters through introducing policies by public authorities for the communities they represent and whose needs they are best placed to know (Ross and Chang, 2012); and
- implementation, where actions and interventions can be taken and planned coherently across an administrative area.

Based on these benefits, agencies and organisations have published health-specific advice to support public health and planning professionals in developing locally led guidance, including on planning healthier places and environments (PHE, 2021) and hot-food takeaways (Sustain, 2019).

Neighbourhood and site-level policy and guidance

There is increasing interest being shown in further devolving planning responsibilities to even smaller geographical scales at the neighbourhood level in order to enable communities to take greater ownership of planning issues and processes. Since 2010, localism approaches have been introduced in planning statutes across the UK nations; this level of planning is known as 'neighbourhood planning' in England, 'local place planning' in Scotland, 'place planning' in Wales and 'community planning' in Northern Ireland.

Communities can have greater power and responsibility to decide the best priorities on which to spend money, rather than the money being spent for them by the local authority. For example, in England, communities can be allocated 25 per cent of money from developers as part of new development, known as the 'neighbourhood share' of the Community Infrastructure Levy. The objective is to encourage and help communities to accommodate the impact of new development, and to strengthen the role and financial autonomy of neighbourhoods to invest in local infrastructure and services to meet needs (HMSO, 2013).

Lessons are still being learnt and advice curated to support planning for health actions at this neighbourhood level. However, there is evidence that such community action may not be benefitting those in more deprived neighbourhoods and areas where planning is most needed to secure healthier and more equitable outcomes. One study found that 35 per cent of neighbourhood plans in England are in the 20 per cent least deprived areas, while just 4 per cent are in the most deprived areas (Lichfields, 2018b).

The benefits of creating a health planning policy requirement at this level are to ensure:

- the ownership of issues and interventions where these would have a direct and specific impact on the wider determinants of health in a locality; and
- accountability and responsibility, including aligning policy to infrastructure investment allocation and spending decisions to fund interventions that make an equitable difference to health outcomes.

Neighbourhood planning for health in Warwickshire

In support of neighbourhood planning groups across the five lower-tier authorities, Warwickshire County Council's Public Health department developed guidance to set out the evidence for the wider determinants of health. These are elements like housing, access to services, education, training and employment that can be tackled through the neighbourhood development planning process in consultation with community groups and housing developers.

Effectiveness of policy on health

Determining whether a health planning policy can be effective, proportionate and implementable is both an art and a science, being based on judgement and hard data. For example, the process is adjudicated against several contextual factors in addition to evidence:

- Procedural: planning law will often set out the mandatory stages of policy development against which draft plans and policies will be adjudicated (or, in English planning jargon, examined in public) by government-appointed professionals before they can be finalised and adopted for implementation. Many health policies fail to pass this stage, resulting in a lighter-touch policy or being deleted altogether. Therefore, it is important that public health professionals are aware of the planning process and associated legal requirements.

• Relational: planners are gatekeepers who determine the priorities for policy development and are key to managing working relationships in order to develop the right type and intensity of policy that is effective and meaningful. This means having public health professionals with the necessary capability to understand the nuances of the language and parameters of planning (Ross and Chang, 2012).

• Impact and outcome based: the use of social, economic and environmental assessments to inform and assess the health impact of policies is often a requirement, particularly across the EU, where human health issues are part of the SEA process. However, research continues to find poor consideration of health in this process (Fischer et al, 2020).

Health planning policy eight-stage process

There is a need for those involved in healthy planning policy development to work together to adopt a clearly defined set of priorities and an integrated approach to planning for health and wellbeing, starting with local representative bodies of the health system to ensure that their investment activities are aligned. An eight-stage health planning policy approach (Figure 7.1) can help bring forward a process that makes planning policies for health effective, meaningful and impactful, and that meets procedural and impact and outcome-based requirements.

Stage 1: Establish capacity

This cross-cutting stage is critical and should form the basis of not only building and developing working relationships with planners and the wider built environment family, but also undertaking the activities set out in the following stages. This

Figure 7.1: An eight-stage health planning policy approach

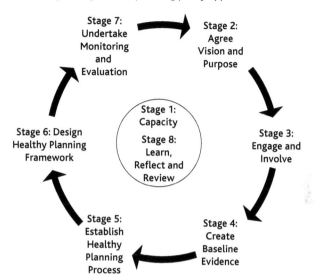

can involve recruiting joint specialist posts, including planning for health in job descriptions and portfolio responsibilities, or organising training and professional development sessions (for further detail, see Chapter 9). This stage should not be seen as standalone, but be integrated as part of an organisation's workforce strategy, or corporate commitment to the agenda.

Stage 2: Agree vision and purpose

There are many perspectives, frameworks, priorities and emphases on what the wider determinants mean locally, so agreeing on a shared vision, priorities and purpose across teams, departments, organisations and stakeholders is important. This can result in a vision statement that all parties can agree to and work from in order to develop healthy planning policies that are mutually beneficial (NHS England, 2019).

Stage 3: Engage and involve

There are many stakeholders and interested parties involved in setting out priorities around the wider determinants, including the communities who will be the ultimate beneficiaries from improved public health outcomes. As explained previously, local policy development processes will already have statutory requirements for public consultation and engagement, and neighbourhood planning processes exist to give communities the power and capacity to create planning policies specific to their needs.

Stage 4: Create baseline evidence

Healthy planning policies should be not only aspirational, but also realistic and deliverable. In order for effective decisions to be made based on the policies, they must be based on adequate, up-to-date and relevant evidence about the social, economic, health and wellbeing needs of the area and the communities. Public health departments will have a wealth of information used to inform commissioning activities (PHE, 2021). Planners need to work with public health departments to understand and take account of such information, as well as any data about environmental barriers/population behaviours to improving health and wellbeing.

Stage 5: Establish a healthy planning protocol

In order to help navigate the legal process of the planning system, establishing a protocol, or way of working, can be a way to support more meaningful public health involvement. This process will set out: who will have vested interests or statutory responsibilities in relation to planning and public health; what information, intelligence and evidence are available; where and how they are best involved in the policy development process; and the means to review and evaluate this working relationship.

Planning for health protocol in Norfolk, England

A protocol was set up in the county of Norfolk to establish a working relationship and simplified processes for using health and social care information to inform plan making and decision-making between Norfolk County Council (where public health functions sit), its eight planning authorities at the lower-tier district levels, relevant health and social care partners, and commissioning bodies.

Stage 6: Design a healthy planning framework

A healthy planning framework will support the operation of the protocol based on an adopted policy or policies. It will set out expectations and seek to align standards for health-related policy areas, such as housing, infrastructure, natural environment and sustainable transport. It can include a self-assessment checklist to review legislative and national policy compliance, which is essential if the policy is to be accepted through procedural checks. Frameworks are adopted as guidance but subordinate to local plans and policies.

Planning for health national policy compliance checklist

A national planning policy compliance checklist was created for England against the NPPF, cross-referenced with the 'National Design Guide' and the 'Planning Practice Guidance', and posed questions for planning and public health officers in developing policy. This was created as part of PHE's 'Getting research into practice' resource by the TCPA and University of the West of England (PHE, 2021).

Stage 7: Undertake policy monitoring and evaluation

There should be a mechanism or process to monitor and evaluate on a regular basis the impact and outcomes of a policy, such as healthy homes. The vision statement created at the start of this process can form a useful reference point. There will often be statutory monitoring requirements for plans and strategies on an annual basis, but governments may not specify what indicators or key performance indicators should be used. For health and wellbeing, there are multiple indicator characteristics:

- indicators that set out progress against health trend data, such as childhood obesity rates, general reported wellbeing or rates of physical activity;
- topic-based indicators with associations made to health outcomes using wider research publications, such as the number of homes built to a specified healthy planning standard, the square metres of public open space provided or the number of cycle parking provided; and
- procedural indicators to track key healthy planning requirements, such as the number of HIAs received.

Stage 8: Learn, reflect and review

This second, cross-cutting stage is critical and linked to the capacity stage. It is about understanding and regularly reflecting on the processes and actions that can and will lead to making positive impact on health and wellbeing. On plans and policies, this may involve regular reviews based on legal requirements (often every five years) or a changing evidential basis. In practice, this can involve holding regular meetings between planning and public health departments to reflect on a particular project or policy activity. This stage should not be seen as standalone, but be integrated as part of an organisation's skills and capacity strategy, or corporate commitment to learning and development.

Concluding statement

Having a strong and explicit policy basis for planning for health should not be underestimated. This chapter has provided an eight-stage process to creating effective and robust healthy planning policies. Having a supportive planning policy or set of policies on public health-related issues is a necessary prerequisite for initiating and justifying action.

8

Health and wellbeing
in planning decisions

> Although public health can be made a material
> consideration in planning decisions, it is sometimes
> a secondary concern.
>
> House of Commons Health
> Select Committee (2018, p 27)

The pace of change across communities is staggering, with the UK government having ambitions to build 300,000 new homes (equivalent in size to the south-west city of Bristol) every year. The scale and scope of such change through new residential and commercial land uses will have impacts on population and individual health and wellbeing.

Once policy frameworks are in place, practitioners have the challenging task of translating them into actionable decisions on proposals that range from the individual home or retail premise to large-scale communities. Often, this starts with the basic question of whether and how public health issues are considered in the planning process. Then, there are questions of how public health professionals are involved in the decision-making process and whether they need to be involved in all decisions given limitations on capacity and resources – unless there is dedicated capability, which is not currently common practice, but does exist in many public authorities, such as Torbay and East Sussex.

This chapter will describe mechanisms to frame understanding of the decision-making relationships between planners and public health teams where planning decisions can constitute public health decisions (Wells et al, 2010):

- the main barriers that decision-makers face when considering health issues in planning;
- how public health issues can be material considerations in the decision-making process, illustrated with practical examples; and
- the 'gateways' or opportunities for public health involvement.

Addressing the barriers

Chapter 3 highlighted the strategic barriers that front-line planning practitioners face, including when making decisions that have implications for a range of public health and wider socio-economic outcomes. This may be due to planners finding it challenging to interpret and apply public health evidence to the varying spatial scales and at a granularity where the evidence needs to be tailored to the particular site subject to planning consent (Carmichael et al, 2019), or where public health professionals are unclear as to how best to contribute to the decision-making process and have a positive effect on the outcome of the decision. Sometimes, due process may not lead to the right outcome for public health. This issue is particularly prominent in a planning system that is 'discretionary', such as that in the UK, and is subject to the professional balancing of policy considerations by planners. It contrasts with a more rigid but certain system based on adherence to specified rules and standards, such as the US, New Zealand or other zoning-based systems.

Who are the decision-makers?

Those with responsibilities for decisions are:

- The government policymaker: the planner and/or civil servant tasked with writing policy requirements at the national level.
- The planning authority planner: the planner making decisions on individual development applications. They will not be the

same as the ones developing the planning policy and strategy, but tasked with implementing them.

- The local planning committee politician: many jurisdictions place the final legal decision-making responsibility on elected politicians sitting on planning committees, who act on the recommendations of the planning authority planner. Which applications are decided by the politician or by the planner will vary from authority to authority.
- The planning appeal case adjudicator: the planning process has a right of appeal, where the planning applicant can appeal against the decision of the planning authority.

Making public health a material consideration in decision-making

A fundamental question was and continues to be whether public health issues are considered in the planning decision-making process. This is a recurring question posed by many in public health departments and pondered by many in planning departments, which can be the source of mistrust, miscommunication and basic misunderstanding.

The answer is not as straightforward as 'yes' or 'no', and it is a constant area of frustration and legal clarifications through the judiciary system. Those working in public health may wonder why there is ambiguity, particularly if a consent application for land uses and building designs may result in people's health and wellbeing being compromised. However, depending on the interests represented, the answer to the question will be based on five factors:

- legal – what the law allows;
- policy – what policy requirements there are to lead to a sound decision;
- procedural – how decisions should be made;
- scale and locality – what locality or site public health issues relate to; and
- professional – what qualified and accredited professionals should do.

Definition of material consideration

From established case law, any consideration that relates to the use and development of land is capable of being a planning consideration. It must relate to the purpose of planning legislation, which is to regulate the development and use of land in the public interest, and fairly and reasonably relate to the application concerned (see Stringer *v* Minister of Housing and Local Government [1970] 1 WLR 1281).

Legal

Planning law will set out: what the parameters are for the purpose of the planning system; the legal functions and responsibilities of the public authority and interested bodies; the objectives the carrying out some functions will achieve; and expected protocols and procedures for decision-making. Such law will range from having a guiding principle that decisions should be made according to localised policy, to setting down specific conditions by which applications will be granted. The degree of specificity and who determines this is important to ensuring that decisions are made in the best interests of the affected persons and their health and wellbeing.

Permitted development rights is a prime example to highlight. This is a dedicated planning consenting system under the Town and Country Planning (General Permitted Development) (England) Order 2015, which allows certain specified developments, often minor and very small-scale in nature, to be built. The process will not require full *local* planning decision-making process, but rather a lighter-touch process based on 'conditions' that are set *nationally*.

For converting from commercial to residential uses, legislation only allows the planning authority to consider conditions relating to: (1) the transport and highways impacts of the development; (2) contamination risks on the site; (3) flooding risks on the site; (4) the impacts of noise from commercial premises on the intended occupiers; and (5) the provision of adequate natural light in all habitable rooms of the dwelling houses. The effect of such a narrow set of conditions to frame decisions on people's living environments can be profound, as wider physical and mental health factors cannot be considered (Marsh et al, 2020).

Permitted development conversions to residential use and health

A planning case in Watford in the south-east of England concerned a proposed conversion from an industrial premise to 15 studio flats. The planning authority refused the initial application on various grounds relating to the poor quality of the living environment, arguing that it 'would have serious impact upon the health of the future occupiers'. During the appeal process, the planning inspector concluded in his judgement that while he recognised that 'the proposed units are small and that, for example, living without a window would not be a positive living environment ... the provisions of the General Permitted Development Order 2015 require the decision makers to solely assess the impact of the proposed development in relation to the conditions.' A decision was made in 2019 to allow the appeal and the development was therefore granted consent to be built. This is a case where the specificity of legislation has had unintended consequences of not allowing other important considerations to be included, thereby creating potential for occupants' health and wellbeing to be compromised.

Policy

Policy requirements set by planning authorities will frame the decisions to be made. This aspect of planning decision-making via policy compliance is particularly critical to note because planning legislation will dictate such a necessity. For example, the English planning legislation, the Town and Country Planning Act 1990, specifies that decisions shall have regard to the provisions of the development plan. The planning authorities' development plan or planning strategy will contain a range of policy requirements, including on health and wellbeing (though not in all authorities), as the TCPA's (2019) policy review of local plans in England and Wales found.

National policy and guidance can also specify how public health issues should be taken into account in the process, which, in turn, can be material considerations. Policies developed in health settings outside the planning system may also be material considerations. These can be policies developed as part of strategies to tackle diseases through prevention, obesity and healthy weight, mental wellbeing, and physical inactivity. For them to be considered material, they need to be relevant to planning and be explicit about planning's contribution and role.

England's NPPF stated the following requirement for healthy communities, and the *italicised* texts can be material when considering planning and health issues:

> Planning policies and decisions should aim to achieve healthy, inclusive and safe places which … enable and support healthy lifestyles, especially where this would address identified local health and wellbeing needs – *for example through the provision of safe and accessible green infrastructure, sports facilities, local shops, access to healthier food, allotments and layouts that encourage walking and cycling.* (MHCLG, 2021b, p 27, para 92c)

However, it should be noted that each nation or planning jurisdiction will have different policy requirements. To ensure a structured and systematic approach to considering these policy requirements relevant to health, planners have worked with public health teams to create planning for health guidance and checklists. Public agencies and VCSE stakeholders have also created such guidance and checklists, and there is a wide-ranging and extensive list of examples used in practice (see Pineo et al, 2018; see also Table 8.1). Often, such a checklist is published as a de facto HIA approach to assist planners and planning applicants to make rapid assessments against local health and wellbeing considerations. Ultimately, the premise is that, first and foremost, a decision must be taken to ensure policy compliance.

Table 8.1: Examples of planning for health guidance, frameworks and checklists

International/country specific	Local/ municipal level	Topic specific	Assessment/ certification
Developed by international and national government bodies or agencies. High level and therefore can be transferrable regardless of country's legislative requirements.	Developed by local authorities based on evidence or good practice. Often adapted from or with reference to variety of other frameworks. These are often adapted as de facto assessment tools for plans and projects.	Developed by VCSE sector bodies and are specific to defined topics or environmental interventions. These are non-statutory in status and therefore have limited weight in decision-making unless adopted into local policy.	Developed as accreditation or certification tools by public or VCSE bodies. Many are referenced in national or local policies, and may not always be oriented to public health outcomes.

Use of a checklist to consider public health issues in Torbay

Torbay, a coastal authority in England's south-west region, developed planning guidance in 2017 called 'Healthy Torbay'. At the heart of the guidance is a 'Torbay healthy planning checklist', which can be used by applicants to consider relevant health and wellbeing issues in Torbay and how they relate to the proposal. The checklist is structured around a series of questions and grouped around four themes: 'travel Torbay', 'healthy homes', 'healthy places' and 'prosperous bay'. It supports the policies contained in the Torbay local plan and can be used in the planning decision-making process.

Procedural

As well as decisions taken with regards to policies in the development plan, the other component of the legislation is the role of additional material considerations in the process. These

Table 8.2: Examples of material and non-material planning considerations relevant to health and wellbeing

✓ Material issues	X Non-material issues
Government policy, guidance, ministerial statements and so on	Matters controlled under non-planning legislation
Loss of sunlight	Private issues between neighbours
Overshadowing/loss of outlook to the detriment of residential amenity	Loss of view
Overlooking and loss of privacy	Problems arising from construction
Highway and traffic impact	Strength or volume of local opposition
Capacity of physical infrastructure	Opposition to business competition
Deficiencies in local facilities	Loss of property value
Incompatible or unacceptable uses	
Layout and density of building design	

considerations must be planning related, and established practice and case law from the courts have determined what are or are not material planning considerations (see Table 8.2). Balancing the weight of considerations in determining an application is at the discretion of the decision-maker and will often fall within the responsibility of an individual town planner in charge of the casework.

Public health issues can be material considerations, but how these issues are framed in relation to planning and development, and determining their materiality, can be achieved through public health involvement. For developments of a certain size, there will be requirements to undertake an EIA and submit an EIA report as part of the application process. Planners will then consider the report with other assessment reports before deciding on the outcome. For public health, EU regulations on EIA require consideration of population and human health factors. Many applications that do not fall within EIA requirements may be subject to HIA requirements set by local planning authorities. However, unless HIA is a legal requirement, such as in Wales through the Public Health (Wales) Act 2017, or articulated as policy requirements, assessing health issues will not be an automatic default action by planners (for further details on HIA and EIA requirements, see Part II of this book).

As a matter of principle, there is no reason why public health professionals within the same public authority or from other sectors and organisations should be prevented from participating in the decision-making process. Good practice and law will often encourage, if not require, public and expert consultation to take place before a decision is made. Legislation or policy may also specify which stakeholders will have a statutory right to be consulted. For example, according to the Infrastructure Planning (Prescribed Consultees and Interested Parties etc.) (Amendment) Regulations 2021, for strategic and large-scale infrastructure projects in England, such as power stations, motorways, waste treatment plants and airport developments, the UK Health Security Agency is required by legislation to be consulted where applications 'could potentially cause harm to people and are likely to affect significantly public health'.

Many planning departments will include the local public health department or a strategic public health agency as a non-statutory consultee. This provides the opportunity for public health involvement and input from public health evidence and needs assessments into the decision-making process. Furthermore, in the UK, there is the opportunity in the preliminary stages of an application process before formally submitting the application for 'pre-application' discussions with the public authority planning department. Similarly, the opportunity exists in the appeals process, which is an emerging research focus on public health issues (O'Malley et al, 2021). Often, planning departments will seek to involve public health teams if it is appropriate and relevant to do so.

In addition to the procedures required by law, each public authority will have its own process for decision-making by the relevant accountable officers or committees. This is a process in which public health professionals can have multiple opportunities to engage with planners (TCPA, 2015). It is also during this process where it can best be determined whether issues are material or non-material. Ultimately, there needs to be a recognition that due process of public health involvement may not result in a desirable public health decision given the range of other stakeholder views and material considerations that planners will need to consider and balance.

Fast-food restaurant approved despite obesity concerns

A fast-food drive-through restaurant planning application was submitted in a Nottinghamshire district of Mansfield in 2019. The upper-tier health authority in Nottinghamshire County Council objected to the application, citing childhood obesity as a major local public health challenge for Nottinghamshire and the location of the drive-through, with its close proximity to three primary schools. While the planning authority had a hot-food takeaways exclusion zone policy, the proposal lay outside of the exclusion zone. The planning officer recommended granting permission on the basis that the Council do not have any policy reasons to object to the proposed development on health grounds and/or the impact upon local school children. However, the final decision-makers were the politicians on the Planning Committee, who refused the application on public health grounds. The decision was taken to appeal and the public health issue was the main reason for the appeal. However, the planning inspector agreed with the planning officer's assertion that there would be an 'expectation that children of a primary school age would be accompanied by a parent or guardian who would be reasonably expected to have a child's health in mind when selecting meal choices'. The application was granted in 2021.

Scale and locality

As noted previously, planning is undertaken at various geographical scales, over different spatial locations and as regards diverse types of land-use activities. What and how public health issues are considered will and should be very different in a rural locality with proposed standard residential dwellings than in a metropolitan centre with mixed land-use activities for a student population. These are the varieties and permutations planners face day to day in decision-making, and there is a need for public health involvement and tailored evidence to be made applicable to support and aid the process.

Often, public health involvement will be prioritised for developments with significant health impact given limitations on time and resources to respond to all planning applications. For example, a large-scale 200-home residential community will command more attention than a single commercial food retail unit. This is understandable from a project management and capacity planning perspective. From a public health perspective, the scale of land-use activity is sometimes not the only contributing determinant of health; rather, the epidemiology of the relationship between the land-use activity and the affected population is important.

Unsustainable housing scheme refused in Bridgend

In the borough of Bridgend in South Wales, an application was submitted for 41 affordable residential homes. The decision-making process referred to 'Planning Policy Wales' (Welsh Government, 2021a) and the national sustainable place-making outcome of facilitating accessible and healthy environments. This contributed to the refusal of the scheme in 2018 by the planning authority based on material considerations of noise impact and the effect on the living conditions and future wellbeing of adjacent residents and the future occupiers of the proposed housing, as well as the lack of suitable walking, cycling and public transport facilities, meaning that future residents would be dependent on private cars. The applicant appealed the decision and then lost in 2020.

Developing a planning and health protocol is an approach undertaken by public authorities to help determine public health involvement. These protocols are often linked to whether an HIA may be required. Such triggers can be based on the following:

- Size: the scale of development, for example, defined in terms of dwellings (10 or more dwellings are classified as major developments), area coverage (over 0.5 hectares, floorspace of over 1,000 m^2) and significant or strategic infrastructure projects.

- Land use: activities that can be at greater risk and vulnerable to the impact of development on public health outcomes, such as educational, health and social care services, leisure or community meeting settings, food and betting shop retail, and older people or retirement housing.
- Location: sites in areas of high deprivation, with fuel poverty, noise or air pollution, elderly or vulnerable groups, or poor health outcomes based on published and up-to-date health statistics.

Professional

Should the application proceed even if there is the potential for wellbeing harm to the occupants from excessive noise or air pollution but there are other benefits and it is permitted within policy parameters? These may be some of the ethical dilemmas facing planners making decisions or representing clients, as well as those public health professionals being consulted on proposals.

Despite working to organisational or corporate expectations as employees, qualified planners and public health professionals individually adhere to codes of ethical conduct and competencies set out by their representative professional bodies. Whether public health issues are relevant to planners is a question that can be explained by referring to the ethics of professional conduct.

Those practising as a planner or public health practitioner should be subject to a code of conduct that requires consideration of public health, population health and equality. Other built environment and health professionals, such as transport planners, architects, landscape architects, environmental health officers or building engineers, should be subject to similar codes to apply their skills and experience to improve public interest outcomes.

Aligning with individuals' professional conscience, as well as personal interest, can be a positive approach to raising the planning for health issue higher up the policy agenda. This is often observed in those localities or organisations and authorities with a more progressive public health spatial planning practice beyond just meeting regulatory and policy directives. However, there are challenges to enforcing positive actions in making decisions to improve health based on professional ethical practice alone:

- codes of ethics apply to individual practice, not the system, so professionals may feel constrained by the system parameters they are legally required to work within;
- professional accreditation is attributed to the individual, not the public authority or organisation they work for; and
- not all practising planners or public health professionals will be accredited for a variety of personal or financial reasons, or are in the process of being accredited, so the code of conduct may not readily apply.

Professional workforce code of conduct

Town planners

Qualified town planners in the UK are accredited by the RTPI. The RTPI was established in 1914 and received a royal charter in 1959. Its royal charter objective is to 'advance the science and art of planning (including town and country and spatial planning) for the benefit of the public'. Under ethics and professional standards advice (RTPI, 2017), members are required to address ethical challenges and to weigh up these challenges in order to come to a professional decision.

Public health workforce

The Faculty of Public Health is the professional standards body for public health specialists and practitioners. Its 'Good public health practice framework' applies to those practising under the domains of health improvement, health protection and healthcare public health. Practitioners have a 'duty to monitor, protect and improve the health of populations', including investigating and acting on risks to health and poor outcomes in particular populations, or providing professional advice to others on emerging health issues (FPH, 2016).

Concluding statement

There is a need for planners to view public health issues in the decision-making process as a matter of course, not a choice or discretion, and not simply be reliant on the input of public health professionals in the process. Conversely, the need for public health involvement in the process can help planners make more informed and evidence-based decisions to meet local health needs and challenges.

Built environment professionals need to appreciate the long history and foundations of town planning that emerged from concerns about the public's health and sanitation, and have confidence and trust in the planning system and due process. One UK director of public health acknowledged that 'Planners have been trained to think about health impacts – it might not be called that but it is part of what you do when you're a town planner' (TCPA, 2012, p 15). We can instil confidence and trust in each other's professionalism and expertise, but this must be demonstrated through the decisions we make in planning to protect and promote health.

Addendum: more examples of planning decisions

Sustainable community approved in Cambridgeshire

A new town of up to 6,500 new homes in Waterbeach in the East England county of Cambridgeshire was proposed in 2017 and granted planning permission in 2019. As part of the application, an HIA was submitted, as required by South Cambridgeshire District Council policy and supplementary guidance. The HIA was framed around a set of health and wellbeing objectives that the HIA consultant based on the determinants for health set out in national guidance and strategies, including healthy homes, active travel, pollution and environmental risk, and community wellbeing.

Healthy new town homes approved in Darlington

An application of 81 homes was submitted in the North-East England town of Darlington in 2017. The site formed part of Darlington's involvement in the NHS Healthy New Towns (HNT) programme as a demonstrator site. The Darlington HNT design principles informed the masterplanning of the proposal, including meeting Lifetime Homes Standards. While the planning authority did not have specific policies on health and wellbeing, and did not receive consultation feedback from the public health teams during the decision-making process, a range of material considerations informed the decision, including the HNT principles, green spaces, residential amenity and transportation. The application was granted approval in 2017.

Hot-food takeaways applications refused in South Tyneside

In the north of England, there were two separate planning applications for hot-food takeaways in 2020. The public health department objected to the applications, highlighting local health and obesity prevalence. Interestingly, the planning authority did not have a planning policy on public health, though had a policy on managing hot-food takeaways. However, the authority did have supplementary planning guidance on hot-food takeaways and health, adopted in 2017, which contributed to planning officers' decisions to refuse the planning applications on public health grounds. This is an example of where public health involvement, supported by policy and guidance, can be effective in making healthy planning decisions.

Special needs school approved despite poor design

A new school building application in Sutton, South London, was submitted in 2019. The proposed building was a four-storey building, creating a new secondary school and special educational needs school. The planning authority refused the application on grounds including the poor quality of design and internal layouts, but the application was appealed. The planning inspector agreed and recognised that the 'main school would include roughly 16 internal classrooms, that would not have natural light' but argued that mitigating measures could be introduced, such as timetabling to ensure that no child or teacher would spend prolonged periods of time in classrooms with no natural light or view to the outside. He determined that given the small number of affected classrooms, the proposed scheme would provide a high-quality learning and teaching environment. The application was approved in 2020.

Change of housing use with resulting safeguarding concerns for vulnerable persons

An application for a change of use from office to residential was submitted in Lewis, East Sussex, for studio flats and a two-bedroom flat for private rented accommodation. The housing was approved in 2016 under permitted development, so the council could only consider traffic impact, flooding and noise. It has since been used by a neighbouring council for temporary emergency housing. Healthwatch East Sussex independently reviewed the housing block in 2021 and recommended it should not house vulnerable residents.

9

Rise of the public health spatial planning practitioner

> The power wielded by planners in national, regional and local governments to reduce disease and promote wellbeing is the subject of growing awareness, yet there are many unrealised opportunities to ensure the profession can more fully achieve these aims as part of core planning competencies and activities.
>
> Pineo et al (2021, p 75)

The professional workforce is the driving force behind planning for health. Public sector managers and political leadership recognise the importance of having the capacity and capability to work more effectively to influence decisions on policy and planning applications. Private sector directors recognise the financial win–win of investing in the upskilling and reorientation of the workforce to maximise the potential of the market in wellbeing/wellness in urban developments. In areas without a history of joint working, this means starting from scratch and learning the completely new language of planning for health. Driven by the impact of COVID-19, as well as in the years leading up to 2019, there is a new craving for professionals competent in public health spatial planning practice.

This chapter will capture the emerging pivotal role of public health spatial planners in bridging professional boundaries and the training, education and job descriptions necessary to upskill the future generations of the workforce. It builds on established respective planning and public health skills and competency frameworks (see Chapter 2), with shared responsibilities as ambassadors of the profession to ensure that activities are undertaken for the benefit and protection of population health and wellbeing. This chapter will highlight:

- the dedicated practitioner;
- the public health practitioner with a wider determinants of health portfolio;
- the professionally accredited practitioner; and
- the state of current education and professional development.

Who is the public health spatial planning practitioner?

It should be noted that, in many ways, planning for health should and is becoming a way of practice of all professionals, not just planners and public health specialists. Having a workforce that reflects the population being planned for and whose health is being protected and improved upon means ensuring that workforce planning achieve a balanced workforce that is fit for purpose and has diverse demographic characteristics and life and professional experiences. The RTPI has recognised the need to improve diversity and inclusion in the planning profession, whose current membership is 61 per cent male and includes only 6 per cent from black, Asian and minority ethnic groups. Ultimately, a more representative workforce will help practitioners obtain the range of competencies needed.

Practitioners originating from multiple 'home' disciplines are identified as working in planning for health, including environmental health officers, architects, landscape architects, building services engineers and environmental managers. Their practice or job descriptions will share the type of necessary skills, competencies and working knowledge required in understanding spatial planning and the public health systems or outcomes. In this regard, the practitioner can be considered as a standalone role consolidating expertise and capacity, or part of many roles sharing and spreading capability (see Figure 9.1).

While the single term 'practitioner' is used, in practice, responsibilities may reside in one single post or be shared across

Figure 9.1: The interdisciplinary public health spatial planning practitioner

Public health spatial planning practitioner

Spatial planning expertise

Public health expertise

Interdisciplinary practitioners

Urban design

Building services engineer

Healthcare

Landscape architect

Planning

Transport

Community development

Property developer

Public health

Environmental health

Sustainability

Surveyor

Architect

Impact assessor

Housing

Multiple 'home' disciplinary practitioner

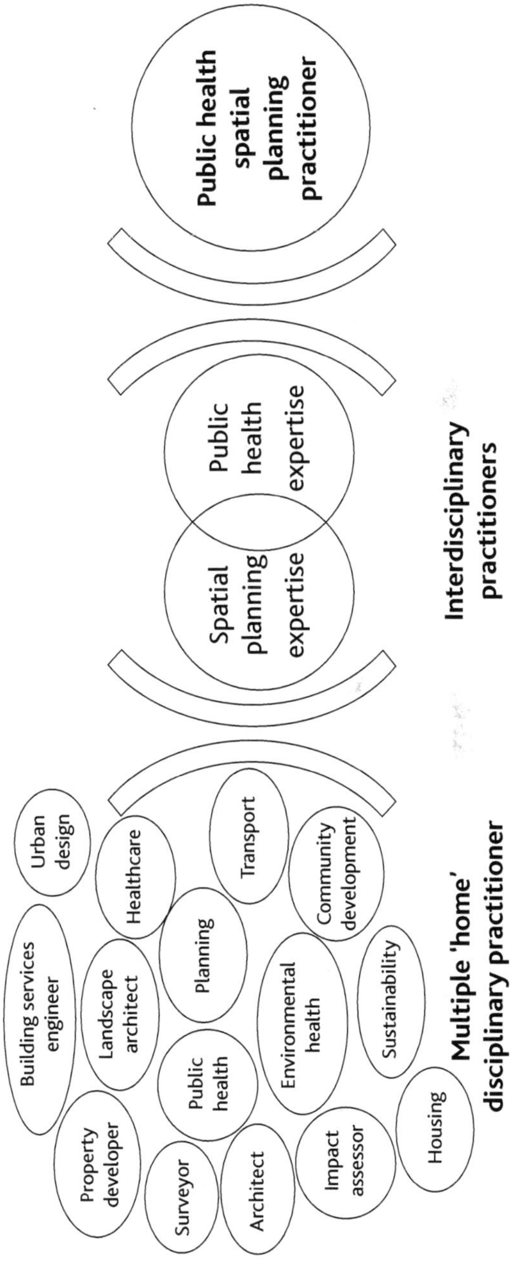

Table 9.1: Pros and cons of dedicated role versus shared responsibilities of a public health spatial planning practitioner

	Pros	Cons
Dedicated practitioner role	1. Specific additional capacity proportional to priority setting. 2. Consolidation of expertise to maximise impact. 3. Not prone to reassignment or reprioritisation of work. 4. Statement of shared commitment between teams if role is jointly funded. 5. Act as leader/champion to drive change and impact.	1. Lack of sufficient pool of expertise of the role. 2. Overreliance on individuals without wider acquisition/transfer of knowledge. 3. Prone to excessive workload or prioritisation of work. 4. Complete loss of momentum if role changes/ceases. 5. Pressure and sustainability of staffing budget.
Shared practitioner roles	1. Ability to share workload and responsibilities when needed. 2. 'Multiplier' effect of transfer of knowledge across teams. 3. Statement of aligned commitment between teams. 4. Working example of HiAP approach.	1. Prone to conflict if one team management/priority changes. 2. Prone to reprioritisation if one or more shared roles or individuals change. 3. Reliance on agreed working arrangement between teams. 4. Temporary loss of momentum due to one or more shared roles or individuals changing.

multiple roles in the public authority or organisation, with pros and cons of each approach (see Table 9.1). Decisions taken to share capability and/or increase capacity on the payroll will follow good practices on workforce planning (CIPD, 2020). They are often based on the following factors:

• Contribution to priorities: what is the organisational, departmental or team priority for planning and health in the context of any legislative or policy requirements, the duration of such requirements, and the degree of need to justify needing the practitioner?

- Impact on budget and resources: what resources and opportunities are there to either increase the staff headcount or share responsibilities across different roles and grades of the role, or over the duration of the commitment? And what is the degree of impact of both options on achieving outcomes?
- Access to existing and readily available (external and internal) expertise: is there the opportunity to draw on wider expertise through external consultant contracting, temporary placements or shared roles across teams or organisations.

There is a golden thread: spatial planning's and the practitioner's ability to apply and implement interdisciplinary planning for health skills, knowledge and competencies through influencing spatial planning's policy development and decision-making processes.

Who is the public health spatial planning practitioner?

Dedicated practitioner

A dedicated additional post for planning and health is created mainly in the public sector, such as in a central government agency or local authority. It is considered part of a team or leading an HiAP approach to healthy places by having or developing expertise in planning, housing, environment and transport. This leadership role is critical to help maintain and increase the reach and visibility of the planning and health agenda at national or more local levels, especially if such a role is a rarity.

Responsibilities of the post will involve providing technical advice to the public health and planning teams on actions to improve health and wellbeing, including policy development. Responsibilities will also include supporting the implementation of programmes and coordinating the public health response to planning applications for urban development projects, such as housing, transport or utilities infrastructure. It can be jointly funded or solely funded by one department. While the role will straddle two or more departments, the primary home department would often be public health, which is indicative of the need to have obtained public health skills and competencies, or their equivalent.

The contents of a job description will often include, among other things:

- providing expert or specialist input subject to regulatory or policy requirements;
- providing evidence and supporting the analysis of evidence to ensure that the health needs of the community are represented and advocated for;
- identifying and supporting opportunities to embed health and wellbeing outcomes into economic, infrastructure and built environment initiatives and workstreams, and managing the development of options where appropriate;
- leading the coordination of public health responses to planning application consultations, including gathering data, writing reports and undertaking HIAs;
- creating bespoke formatted planning for health templates and frameworks;
- supporting the development of relationships with planning teams to enhance the public health influence across the system, including delivering of training and professional development activities;
- providing a contact and liaison point for other teams that need to discuss the public health approach in relation to wider determinants; and
- identifying, developing and maintaining good working relationships with internal and external colleagues.

Creating a dedicated post in the local authority is one of the recommendations of the TCPA on improving the capacity and capability of public health planners (TCPA, 2019). Since 2019, there are many more local authorities and public agencies creating dedicated posts, which demonstrates the level of political, policy and financial commitment to planning for health.

The public health policy officer

A public health officer role was established in the Public Health Division of the Place and Wellbeing Directorate of a London borough authority. This dedicated post was aimed at someone with built environment or town planning experience who would like to develop professional skills to 'plan for health', or someone with public health experience with an interest in developing knowledge and experience in place making. The wide-ranging job description set out responsibilities according to knowledge, training and experience, including health information, evidence and needs assessment, research, audit and evaluation, commissioning of health and wellbeing and council services, and policy/service development. It was expected that the candidate would be educated at the postgraduate level in public health or the built environment, and have a strong commitment to addressing the wider determinants of health and tackling health inequalities.

Shared practitioner roles with health, planning and a wider determinants portfolio

For most public authorities, sharing responsibilities for planning and health is common practice, particularly for those roles in public health departments. They will have a range of responsibilities, similar to those for a dedicated practitioner role, across the planning process. These are either included in the job description for 'wider determinants' roles or form part of the annual work programmes of individuals with multiple portfolios. As this role is based in public health departments, it only provides the opportunity for those wishing to develop a formal career in public health, albeit with an interest in planning.

For those working in planning departments, experience with encountering these practitioners indicates that responsibilities for health policy are mostly concentrated in the policy development stage, where the individual may be tasked with developing policy and associated guidance on planning and health. It is less common for planners at the decision-making stages of the planning process to be specifically tasked with health because they will be required by law and policy to consider and balance all issues, not just health. This results, in part, in decisions that may not maximise health outcomes, but, on balance, would be acceptable in planning terms. Addressing this will require training and CPD. As this role is based in the planning department, it only provides the opportunity for those wishing to develop a formal career in planning, albeit with an interest in public health.

Accredited practitioner on healthy buildings and places

There is another group of technical specialists, mainly working in the private sector, who are accredited according to the healthy building/development frameworks that they apply independently when designing and assessing development or building projects. These are independent of and in addition to the 'home' professional qualifications that they may have already obtained for membership of a professional institute.

Designers and developers of new homes and buildings have a range of frameworks and accredited practitioners to select from. These include, but are not limited to, the following:

- *WELL accredited professional* (AP): originating in the US, the International WELL Building Institute (IWBI) developed the WELL Building Standard™ in 2014, which uses a series of evidence-based strategies on 10 core concepts to design mainly commercial buildings that enhance health and wellbeing (IWBI, 2020). These 10 concepts are air, water, nourishment, light, movement, thermal comfort, sound, materials, mind and community. Becoming a WELL AP requires passing a closed-book computer-based exam with 100 multiple-choice questions over two hours. Being a WELL AP means that the individual is an expert in applying the WELL Building Standard™. There are more than 16,000 WELL APs internationally.
- *Fitwel ambassador:* Fitwel is a healthy buildings certification originally created in 2017 by the US Centers for Disease Control and Prevention and US General Services Administration. The Center for Active Design is Fitwel's licensed operator. Fitwel certification is available for different property typologies, with evidence-based strategies to address seven health impact categories, such as increases physical activity, reduces morbidity and absenteeism, supports social equity for vulnerable populations, and instils feelings of wellbeing (Center for Active Design, 2020). For individuals

to become a Fitwel ambassador, they are required to pass the introductory ambassador course, consisting of a 60-minute training video and a 50-question, multiple-choice, online exam. Ambassadors can access the Fitwel Portal to review projects for certification. There are more than 2,800 Fitwel ambassadors internationally.

• *Home Quality Mark assessor:* the Building Research Establishment (BRE) developed the Home Quality Mark (HQM) in 2016 to assess the home and its surroundings according to 11 financial, wellbeing, environmental and social categories (BRE, 2018). These 11 categories are: transport and movement; outdoors; safety and resilience; comfort; energy; materials; space; water; quality assurance; construction impacts; and customer experience. Becoming an HQM assessor requires undertaking online training, attending a two-day classroom course and sitting two 90-minute exams at the end of the second day (BRE Academy, no date). There are around 90 HQM assessors. The BRE also has an extensive list of accredited professionals for other BRE quality frameworks that it has developed.

It should be noted that there are also other non-accredited self-assessment healthy building and development frameworks from which urban designers and developers can select and choose to adopt, such as Building for a Healthy Life, the Place Standard tool and the Essex Livewell Development Accreditation.

Work-based learning practitioner role: placements and secondments

Work placements and secondments provide an injection of on-demand capacity and expertise, either from within or from outside the authority or organisation. Due to the variety of ways in which placements and secondments are undertaken, there are questions over its long-term impact, contribution to increasing capability and development of the public health spatial planning practitioner role. The effectiveness of the role will depend on the expertise and competency of the candidate.

There are multiple options and rationales for placement and secondments:

- *Meeting a skills or knowledge gap*: this suits circumstances where the skill or knowledge does not exist within the team or organisation due to a skills shortage or because the skills are generally not held in that sector or discipline, so that it is more appropriate to bring in outside expertise. Public Practice in the UK is an example where their associates, including those with expertise in wellbeing and healthy places, are offered placements in public authorities (Public Practice, 2020).
- *Delivering a time-limited programme of activities*: this suits circumstances where there is a specific activity planned due to policy or corporate commitments that requires additional capacity or skills. For example, Tower Hamlet's HIA officer was placed on a two-year secondment to support the implementation of the authority's planning policy requirement on HIAs (Carmichael and Richmond, 2020).
- *Filling a short-term vacancy*: this suits circumstances where an existing role has been made vacant temporarily due to changing employment or other personal circumstances.
- *Supporting internships*: this suits organisations with an internship programme or a programme to host and support the training pathway of public health professionals (for an example of PHE's Healthy Places team, see the following box).

Public health registrars on placement in PHE

UK public health registrars are required to undertake a range of public health-based placements as part of their multi-year training pathway to become a public health consultant or specialist. They are required to demonstrate their training against relevant public health competencies frameworks, most notably, the UK Public Health Skills and Knowledge Framework. PHE's Healthy Places team had registrars on regular placement to lead on or support specific activities like research and evidence gathering, stakeholder engagement, and management (for an example, see Insider story 9.2 by Dr Rachael Marsh and Carolyn Sharpe).

Education and professional development

The composition of the workforce is a reflection of its evolutionary journey in education and learning systems. This proposition is put forward to further discussion about the involvement of educators in taking action. Future practitioners should be engaged and upskilled through education before and as they develop their careers in the industry.

The planning for health agenda is neither a novelty nor a recent evolutionary milestone. Much of the previous and continuing engagement in this agenda is through environmental health professionals, but they have a narrower focus on such issues as environmental hazards than on the wider environment, health improvement and inequalities.

The integration of planning and public health in policy and professional terms has only been evident in the last 15 to 20 years. It is true that planners and public health professionals will share similar skills and competencies when undertaking activities in the planning system, as illustrated by a PHE (2020a) case study comparing a planning activity against the competency frameworks of the RTPI (for planners) and the Public Health Skills and Knowledge Framework (for public health professionals).

Their knowledge base and learning journey have been and continue to be completely different, though there is evidence of closer alignment of and convergence towards shared education and development. There is no doubt that professionals should be competent in their 'home' disciplinary skills before they develop a specialism in planning for health. Therefore, in this regard, this chapter focuses on tertiary education at the postgraduate level and CPD approaches.

Tertiary education

Universities, technical colleges and higher education institutions play a critical role in developing the knowledge professionals need and supplementing the further knowledge and skills that both professionals and society demand to meet changing trends and challenges. Most importantly, they play a critical role in

Table 9.2: Summary of pros and cons of approaches to planning for health competencies in university education

	Pros	Cons
Joint specialist masters	Provides a coherent learning reference point to obtain shared knowledge from both schools of planning and public health	Requires students to be competent in both systems, which may not meet expectations or interests
Specialist masters	Allows concentration on a technical specialism or particular aspects of planning and health	Overly specialist on aspects, which may narrow career development opportunities
Standalone elective modules	Allow flexibility to meet students' varying interests and introduce them to more accessible bite-sized learning materials	May not provide the necessary coherent and depth of learning needed to obtain a wider range of skills and competencies

ensuring such skills and knowledge are relevant to and based on the experiences of those in practice.

However, the challenge and dilemma faced by educators is whether to introduce strategic and high-level materials or to tailor the learning to the specific legislative and policy frameworks of the particular country or countries. The formal learning journey provides a structured, safe learning environment to explore, challenge and innovate as the policy landscape is in constant political evolution. Much of the information contained in this book about improving the practice of public health spatial planning is technical and about implementation, not about why planning and health is needed or not. Knowing what to do, how to do it, when to do it and who needs to do what should form the educational basis on mastering the art and science of public health spatial planning.

A scoping review by the authors of a sample of programmes available on public health spatial planning from universities in the UK and US provides an interesting starting point (see Table 9.2). The review identified and broadly distinguished varying approaches to delivering public health spatial planning education and the pros and cons of each.

Through an initial identification of available courses in Table 9.3, there is clearly a geographical and educational divide,

Table 9.3: Examples of postgraduate programmes with specific planning and public health module contents

Joint specialist masters	Harvard Graduate School of Design (USA)	Master in Urban Planning and Master in Public Health
	University of California, Berkeley (USA)	Master of City Planning and Master of Public Health
	University of Illinois (USA)	Master of Public Health and Master of Urban Planning
	University of Buffalo (USA)	Master of Urban Planning and Master of Public Health
	University of Michigan (USA)	Master of Urban and Regional Planning/Public Health
	University of Minnesota (USA)	Master of Public Health and Master of Urban and Regional Planning
Specialist masters	University College London (UK)	MSc Health, Wellbeing and Sustainable Buildings
	University of Derby (UK)	MSc Environmental Health
Standalone elective module	University College London (UK)	MSc Health, Wellbeing and Sustainable Buildings – Health and Wellbeing in Cities: Theory and Practice
	University of Dundee (UK)	MA Urban Planning – People and Places
	University of Sheffield (UK)	MA Urban Design and Planning – Health, Wellbeing and the Built Environment
	University of the West of England (UK)	MSc Urban Planning – Healthy Cities
	Ulster University (UK)	MSc Planning and City Resilience – Healthy Communities
	University of California, Berkeley (USA)	Master of City Planning – Healthy Cities

with the US embracing joint masters, while the UK advances the elective modular offer as part of specialist standalone masters. Further research and engagement with degree programme coordinators will be needed to evaluate the different approaches and their impact on practice and employment opportunities.

CPD

CPD activities fulfil professionals' on-demand requirements and thirst for new and improved skills and knowledge. Outside formal learning through university degrees or courses, CPD is the most effective, and sometimes the only, way to upskill the existing workforce on:

- gaining or refreshing foundational knowledge on the planning system, health system, their relationship and evidence of the impact of this relationship on outcomes;
- raising awareness of emerging trends and challenges on topics, such as an ageing population, health equity and inequalities;
- providing clarity and advice on existing or new legislative and policy requirements; and
- exposing and opening opportunities for networking and contacts with other professionals or professions that would otherwise not be possible.

Professional institutes will publish CPD guidance to direct their membership to undertake, reflect on and report their CPD activities. Maintaining membership of any professional institute requires completing specified hours of CPD in any given year. For example, the RTPI requires 50 hours over a two-year period, while the Faculty of Public Health requires 50 credits or hours in one year (FPH, 2020). Most organisations recognise the need for continuing improvement and will support and actively encourage their employees to allocate working hours to undertake CPD.

'Continuing professional development' is an all-encompassing term that captures all forms of structured or non-structured learning, including placements and secondments. Practitioners should take advantage of the exposure to different ways to obtain and exchange knowledge. The most common CPD activity is

Table 9.4: Examples of CPD activities on planning and public health

Bespoke conferences	• Healthy City Design International Congress, October 2021 • Landscape Institute, 'Health, Wellbeing and Place: How Landscape Delivers Positive Change', January 2021 • Westminster Health Forum, 'Developing Healthy New Towns', June 2018
General conferences with planning and public health content	• RTPI, 'The Planner Live Online', June 2020 • PHE Annual Conference, September 2019 • American Planning Association National Planning Conference (NPC), April 2019
Short CPD 'masterclasses'	• RTPI, 'Planning for Public Health and Wellbeing', May 2021 • Urban Design London, 'Healthy Places', March 2021 • TCPA, 'The 20-Minute Neighbourhood: Learning from Down Under', October 2020 • Health and Wellbeing in Planning Network, 'Planning White Paper and Public Health: Explained', September 2020 • South West Public Health Development School, 'Planning and Health – We Have Enough Evidence; Do We Have Enough Leadership?', October 2019

attending conferences, events, workshops or masterclasses in person or online. Due to the flexible nature of providing and accessing CPD, a range of organisations and sectors provide practitioners with a significant degree of choices. Whether the CPD events are useful is for practitioners to determine as they reflect on learning completion. Table 9.4 shows examples of CPD activities.

Concluding statement

The role, qualifications and experience of the public health spatial planning practitioner is varied, and this chapter has demonstrated that this journey can be a standalone one or integrated. This is positive because it means that planning for health penetrates multiple sectors, disciplines and professions. However, this is also negative because it is a diffusion of knowledge and expertise, and leads to the lack a coherent community of professionals or talent pool to draw from. This underlines the need for a diverse workforce with different backgrounds and life and professional experiences that is more conducive to upskilling in order to incorporate the range of competencies needed for effective public health spatial planning.

Insider story 9.1: Planning, health and sustainability practitioner in Stockport, England

Angie Jukes was Stockport Council's Technical Policy and Planning Officer and shares her experience integrating planning, health and sustainability across the Council. Angie worked at Stockport Council from 2008 until December 2021 as a bridge between planning and public health. Her environmental background and skills informed the links between health and planning. Angie's mantra was "If it doesn't protect and benefit human health, then it isn't sustainable development."

In the middle of the last decade of the 20th century, Stockport Council made a decision to create a unique post. Stockport is a predominantly prosperous borough but has pockets of deprivation and health inequalities that are a major concern. The director of public health coordinated with the Planning Policy Team at Stockport Council to co-fund a post that would deliver sustainability appraisal for the local plan (alongside other statutorily required appraisals and assessments), coordinate the annual policy-monitoring work and promote sustainable design and construction.

In 2008, Angie took over that role and picked up on the work of her predecessors, where they sought to embed health considerations (as part of wider sustainability work) into planning policy. She completed an HIA as part of the statutory sustainability appraisal on the core strategy, followed by work on other draft elements of the local development framework until work began on the new Stockport local plan in 2017.

Angie coordinated the annual planning policy-monitoring work and wrote the annual reports. In addition, she provided guidance to planning officers and applicants on sustainable design and construction. This included health considerations, as outlined in Stockport's 'Sustainable design and construction supplementary planning document', published in 2012. From 2013, she coordinated a 'healthy planning group' of public health and transport colleagues to comment on major applications.

As an environmental professional, she was attracted to the work at the council, as it was committed to reflecting environmental considerations in planning work that would also benefit human health. She had always felt that humans are part of the ecosystem rather than outside of it. Green messages about 'saving the planet' distract from the impacts on our own species. It is human civilisation that is under threat and work to address that must take account of how society works.

The unique approach to sustainability appraisal at Stockport, where a non-planner embedded in the team led the appraisal work, allowed a strong working relationship to be built between planners and the appraiser. However, it also enabled an independence in the appraisal due to links with the director of public health and their individual duty to protect public health. Having a succession of public health leads who understood the importance of biodiversity (especially biophilia) and carbon reduction to human health had been critical in achieving impact over the years.

The review of the existing HIA process to appraise Stockport's core strategy (adopted in 2011) allowed a greater understanding for all stakeholders. This robust process informed wider sustainability appraisal, capturing concerns about health inequalities, an ageing population, static levels of obesity in Stockport's children and health drivers to protect dwindling urban green spaces.

In 2012, the co-writing of a 'Sustainable design and construction supplementary planning document' enabled the capture of health benefits from environmentally sustainable design. The business case for sustainable design and construction also made a clear economic argument for this approach, well before the current shift in economic thinking.

As a result of this work, it was identified that there was a benefit from public health issues informing the planning decision-making process. The head of planning and the director of public health agreed to the establishment of a 'healthy planning group'.

Angie's role was to coordinate comments from public health and transport colleagues on major applications. The process established reflects consideration of the numbers of major applications received per month, alongside the capacity of officers involved. The comments covered wider sustainability, active travel (sustainable transport), green (and blue) infrastructure, affordable housing, age-friendly design and, more recently, suicide prevention, as well as design guidance for care homes (especially infection prevention and control). The comments specifically highlighted the health benefits of these aspects of design and construction. Training was provided to officers to enable them to understand the constraints of the commentary process in planning terms.

Over time, the planners have realised the value of public health comments. Conversely, public health practitioners have gained a greater understanding of the constraints and pressures that planners operate under, as well as the opportunities to influence that work. As a bridge between two highly pressurised professions, Angie was able to inform planning decisions to deliver truly sustainable development across the borough.

Further information

Stockport Council's sustainable development work is available at: www. stockport.gov.uk/sustainable-development

Insider story 9.2: Public health practitioners' viewpoint on planning for health work placement experience

Dr Rachael Marsh and Carolyn Sharpe were public health practitioners undertaking training as public health registrars and on time-limited placements with PHE's Healthy Places team during 2020. They set out distinct skills relevant to planning for health and illustrated the application of these skills in two case-study examples of projects undertaken by Carolyn and Rachael, respectively, while on placement.

They identified five skills sets as core for a practitioner, each of which is relevant to supporting planning systems to create healthy places:

• *Gathering, synthesising and presenting data*: practitioners have the ability to collate, analyse, interpret and communicate qualitative and quantitative data (often using software such as Excel, Nvivo, Stata and SPSS) to both lay and expert audiences. This can include population predictions and modelling scenarios. They are comfortable with national, regional and local routine data sets, and can advise on how to collect bespoke data and appraise data validity and reliability.

• *Systematically reviewing evidence*: practitioners can systematically identify, appraise the quality of and summarise the evidence base in order to consider policy and intervention options, create evidence-informed recommendations, build consensus where there are gaps in evidence and/or advise on further research required.

• *Working and consulting with stakeholders*: practitioners understand which stakeholders need to be engaged on a topic and how to engage them in order to influence an agenda. They are comfortable engaging both internal and external stakeholders, including the public, and consulting with them on challenging and contentious topics when required. They are able to help access groups of the population who do not always have their views represented, such as young people, people with disabilities and minority ethnic groups.

• *Developing, implementing and evaluating policy and programmes*: practitioners can apply the preceding skills in the development and implementation of evidence-based policies and programmes. This can be achieved by ensuring new policies and programmes are monitored and evaluated using routine and bespoke qualitative and quantitative data.

• *Understanding of organisational management and leadership skills*: practitioners can be a public health advocate and leader within their own organisation and across the wider health and planning systems. They can draw on experience of working across disciplines and their understanding of social, cultural and religious perspectives to promote policies and programmes with health, socio-economic and environmental benefits.

Case study: HIA in spatial planning

Carolyn supported the team in developing national and local capability around the use of HIAs. As part of carrying out an HIA, practitioners are required to analyse local qualitative and quantitative data in order to systematically identify the potential health and wellbeing impacts of the plan or planning application, and to assess the potential impacts on health and inequalities. Recommendations to maximise the health and wellbeing benefits and minimise the harm of the plan or planning application should then be developed. When producing recommendations, the practitioner should consult with key stakeholders, including local citizens, developers, health and care professional, and planners. They will also need to draw on the evidence base for spatial planning for health.

The requirement for an HIA to be applied to new plans or planning applications varies by geography. In the UK, as there is no statutory HIA requirement at the national level, HIA policies remain discretionary to local planning authorities. This means that a practitioner would need to work with relevant stakeholders and decision-makers (for example, local planning teams and politicians) to make the case for HIA and advocate for a local HIA policy. In order to add to the evidence base for the effectiveness of HIAs and spatial planning for health, and to draw on lessons learned from the process, it is important for practitioners to monitor and evaluate the extent to which an HIA's recommendations have been taken forward, as well as the actual health and wellbeing impacts of the plan or planning application. Carolyn's work was ultimately published in *Cities & Health* (Sharpe et al, 2021).

Case study: permitted development rights for housing and health

Rachael led on a mixed-methods study of permitted development rights through a systematic review and expert interviews. Permitted development rights constitute a regulatory mechanism in the English planning system that provides automatic permissions for development subject to meeting prerequisite rules. In England, since 2013, the government has been dramatically expanding the role and scope of permitted development rights, despite no assessment of the potential health impacts.

A public health practitioner was able to use many of the skills highlighted earlier to provide the first overview of the health and wellbeing impacts of housing created through permitted development rights. The practitioner's ability to work with stakeholders from multidisciplinary backgrounds enabled engagement with health and planning professionals at the national and local levels on a politically sensitive issue. The practitioner used their understanding of epidemiological principles to create a framework that helped to demonstrate the complex mechanisms through which planning decisions impact on health. Health outcomes, as well as environmental exposures, building features and neighbourhood features, were all included in a systematic evidence review. The practitioner was able to make evidence-informed recommendations for further research and data collection, which are being considered by a national health research funder. They were also able to appraise options for policymakers and propose solutions that appreciate the interdependencies between health, social, environmental and economic outcomes. Rachael's work was ultimately published in *Cities & Health* (Marsh et al, 2020).

Summary

The skill set required by public health practitioners makes them well placed to support the creation of healthy places. Practitioners can be flexible in their approach, and the preceding examples demonstrate how selecting and integrating these skills means that they can be of use for processes at a local level, as well as used for advocating and influencing at a national level.

Further information

Details of training requirements for UK public health registrars are available at: www.fph.org.uk/training-careers/specialty-training

Insider story 9.3: Healthy Development Coordinators: bridging the divide between public health and planning in Tennessee, USA

Dr John Vick is the Evaluation and Assessment Director in the Office of Primary Prevention of the Tennessee Department of Health, and he reflects on the impact of his team of Healthy Development Coordinators. Over the past several years, the Tennessee Department of Health has made substantial investments in built environment initiatives, including new staff, grant funding, technical assistance and educational resources. Key to this work are the department's seven Healthy Development Coordinator positions. Established in 2017, the coordinators support the development of health-promoting environments and policies across the state, serving as connectors between the public health and spatial planning worlds. The positions receive oversight, support and training from the department's Office of Primary Prevention. The department's overall commitment to primary prevention and addressing the root causes of disease led it to grow its built environment work.

The idea for the Healthy Development Coordinator positions arose from a strategic planning process held in 2015 to identify how the department could most effectively invest in connecting public health and the built environment. One of the key recommendations was to recognise the importance of hiring local staff dedicated to engaging with planners and other built environment professionals who understood the unique culture, needs and priorities of each community. Many land-use planning decisions are made at the local level, requiring multiple positions across the state to ensure that the Department of Health can engage in those decisions.

Jurisdiction

Tennessee is divided into 95 county jurisdictions, with the six largest metropolitan areas, including Nashville and Memphis, funding their own local health departments. The remaining 89 counties each have a local health department staffed by the state Department of Health, grouped into seven regional health office jurisdictions. The state-funded coordinator positions work primarily in these suburban and rural counties, including small cities and towns. Relationships and partnerships are critical to the success of the positions, and each coordinator lives and works in one of the state's seven health regions.

Scope and activities

While the positions have a primary focus on increasing physical activity, they engage in diverse disciplinary spaces, including land-use planning, transportation, housing, green space, food access and economic development. They have a variety of backgrounds and expertise, including public health, urban and regional planning, anthropology, and outdoor recreation, and most hold a master's degree. Each coordinator works with community partners to identify initiatives to support in their regions, so the types of projects that they engage in simultaneously reflect both health department priorities and the needs of individual communities, and differ among regions. Coordinators generally engage in the following:

- informing local officials on the health impacts of projects and planning decisions;
- sitting on local, regional and state boards and committees;
- participating in local and regional planning efforts;
- cataloguing healthy built environment assets in local communities;
- providing health data to local partners;
- writing grants to fund health-focused built environment initiatives;
- managing the department's Access to Health built environment grants; and
- evaluating built environment grant projects.

The coordinators are currently piloting a more systematic prioritisation process that allows the coordinators to identify the highest-priority projects through community partner surveys and scans of local plans, and then weight them based on community interest, feasibility, equity and the potential magnitude of the health impact.

Successes and lessons learned

The Healthy Development Coordinators have been successful in shaping local planning efforts and in institutionalising built environment work at the Department of Health. The coordinator positions occupy a middle space between public health and spatial planning, having expertise in both. When partnering with planners, they serve as public health representatives, but they also serve as the planning voice within their local public health departments. They can 'speak both languages', so their value and role shifts depending on the context. Simply having these positions demonstrates the importance of the built environment in shaping health and solidifies this as important to contemporary public health practice. Similarly, having dedicated built environment positions in the health department indicates to partners that health is indeed an important consideration in planning and other built environment efforts.

The coordinators have been well received by partners and are now routinely involved in local planning efforts. They lead design charettes, provide education and best practices to local policymakers, and help write grants for health-focused built environment projects. As health department staff, they can be assets when partnering with planners who want to advocate for healthy planning approaches by bringing an additional level of public health credibility to those efforts. They have also been instrumental in the implementation of the health department's Access to Health grant programme, which provides funding to Tennessee communities for publicly accessible health-promoting built environment projects. The grants have funded 239 projects since 2017, including construction, planning, assessment, convening and programming. The coordinators manage and oversee the evaluation of all grants in their regions, which has allowed them to build relationships with grantees that can be leveraged for future partnerships, as well as helping to demonstrate the impact and value of those investments to communities.

Coordinators need to find the balance between providing support for planners and for built environment efforts, and defining a clear and unique role for them as public health experts. Cross-sector partnerships can be delicate, and it is important to complement rather than duplicate existing efforts when working with other disciplines. While the coordinator positions continue to evolve, they have been a resounding success and have shown that there is a substantive role and demand for dedicated public health staff to support planning work at the local level.

Further information

More details about the Healthy Development Coordinators and the Tennessee Department of Health's built environment work is available at: www.tn.gov/health/health-program-areas/office-of-primary-prevention/ redirect-opp/built-environment-and-health.html

PART IV

Health benefits and outcomes

> The consideration of health and wellbeing has had
> little influence in urban design and planning and yet
> it is the people who live in such conurbations who
> will reap the benefits and disbenefits of the urban
> environment.
>
> RCEP (2007)

Much of the existing literature and investment modelling
seems to corroborate the general view that high-quality and
good design, which is a trait that one would associate with the
outcomes of healthy places and environments, adds economic
value that can be quantified in monetary terms. But is it clear
who pays and who benefits, and when the costs and benefits are
realised and accrued in the planning and development system?

Those working in national and local governments want to
create places in which their populations can live healthier, more
active and more equitable lives. To achieve this, particularly in
more market-led property economies, they need to have the
right policies in place and make the best decisions, as set out in
the previous chapters. However, this alone is not enough; they
also need to engage with the developers, housebuilders and
investors who finance and build those places. They realise that
to achieve healthier places, they need a deeper understanding of
the drivers of investment decisions and the commercial context
in which developers operate when creating new developments
or regenerating established places. They also need to have an
understanding of how legislative and policy mechanisms in
planning can be better used to bring forward not only healthier
schemes, but also economically viable ones.

However, the market is sometimes a step ahead of the
system and policy. In order to help harness and accrue value

generated by healthier places and developments, in recent years, many developers, investors and organisations working with the properly market industry have initiated and developed frameworks, standards and accreditation schemes. Sometimes, these are not due to legislative and policy drivers, but simply because healthy places and planning make business sense.

This part of the book enables readers to:

- help communicate who pays, who benefits and the value case for healthy and viable places, including identifying the many established and emerging healthy development frameworks (see Chapter 10); and
- better understand and help identify mechanisms and examples to secure the necessary financial system investment in elements that are health promoting and will help rebalance investment in neighbourhoods (see Chapter 11).

Part IV key takeaways

- Changing the narrative around the multiple benefits of planning for health for public and private interests can establish a stronger consensus and case for taking action.
- Understanding key decision-makers and investors, often not just public authorities, can help to leverage the power of the private sector to generate meaningful change in planning for health practices and outcomes.
- Combining mandatory legislative and policy directives with the voluntary commitment of developers to sustainable and healthy places provides a powerful partnership and agent of change.
- Securing the untapped investment and financial capacity of the private sector can drive improvements in how practitioners implement planning for health in the community.

10

Value and outcomes

We know from a century of public health research that there is a profound connection between the physical realities of our communities and public health outcomes. While not a new link, COVID-19 has focused us on the influential role the built environment plays in determining our health.

Center for Active Design (2021, p 5)

Much of the existing literature and return on investment modelling seem to corroborate the general view that high quality and good design, which are traits that one would associate with the outcomes of healthy places and environments, add economic value which can be quantified in monetary terms. But is it clear who pays and who benefits, and when are the costs and benefits realised and accrued in the planning and development system?

Those working in national and local governments want to create places in which their populations can live healthier, more active and equitable lives. To achieve this, particularly in more market-led property economies, they need to have the right policies in place and make the best decisions as set out in the previous chapters. However, this alone is not enough – they also need to engage with the developers, the housebuilders and investors, who finance and build those places. They realise that to achieve healthier places they need a deeper understanding of the drivers of investment decisions and the commercial context in which developers operate when creating new developments or regenerating established places. Also they need to have an understanding of how legislative and policy mechanisms in planning can be better used to bring forward healthier but also economically viable schemes.

But the market is sometimes a step ahead of the system and policy. In order to help harness and accrue value generated by healthier places and developments, in recent years many developers, investors and organisations working with the properly market industry have initiated and developed frameworks, standards and accreditation schemes. Sometimes these are absent from legislative and policy drivers, but are done simply because healthy places and planning make business sense.

This part enables the readers to:

- help communicate who pays, who benefits and the value case for healthy viable places including identifying the many established and emerging healthy development frameworks (Chapter 10); and
- better understand and help identify mechanisms and examples to secure the necessary financial and system investment in elements which are health-promoting and will help rebalance investment in neighbourhoods (Chapter 11).

The benefits and value

A small but influential study from 1984 revealed that inpatients in a suburban Pennsylvania hospital who had a window view of green spaces rather than a brick wall, spent about one day less in hospital recuperating and required fewer potent pain relievers following surgery. There seemed to be something inherent in the view of the natural environment that aids recovery and rehabilitation (Ulrich, 1984).

Put simply, well-designed public spaces and neighbourhoods that promote access to green spaces have shown people to experience improved levels of mental health, physical fitness and cognitive and immune function, as well as lower mortality rates in general (WHO, 2019). For example, a recent study found that people living within 100 metres of a high density of street trees had a significantly reduced probability of being prescribed anti-depressants. The study concluded that 'unintentional daily contact to nature through street trees close to the home may reduce the risk of depression, especially for individuals in deprived groups' (Marselle et al, 2020, p 1).

The costs of poor planning/design

The costs of poor design on health and wellbeing to individuals and the public purse can be significant if no actions are taken:

- *Housing*: many homes do not meet basic minimum safety standards, with 23 per cent of private rented homes, 16 per cent of owner-occupied homes and 13 per cent of social rented homes not meeting the England Decent Homes Standard (MHCLG, 2020). Poor housing is estimated to cost the NHS £1.4 billion per year. This does not include wider impacts, such as poorer educational results and decreased job prospects, which have been estimated to cost England some £18.5 billion per annum (Garrett et al, 2021).
- *Air quality*: air pollution is estimated to cost the UK around £16 billion a year, largely through health costs (POST, 2014). It is the biggest environmental threat to health in the UK, contributing to between 28,000 and 36,000 deaths a year, with the main sources being transport (especially road transport) and from industry, agriculture and emissions from homes and businesses (PHE, 2019b). Excess delays, accidents, poor air quality, physical inactivity, greenhouse gas emissions and some of the impacts of traffic noise cost urban areas £38–49 billion a year (Cabinet Office, 2009).
- *Access to green spaces*: £2.1 billion per year could be saved in health costs if everyone in England had good access to green space due to increased physical activity in those spaces (PHE, 2020c).
- *Reductions in health inequalities*: it has been estimated that, overall, reducing health inequalities has the potential to save £31–3 billion per year in productivity losses and £20–32 billion per year in lost taxes and higher welfare payments (Marmot et al, 2010). The Institute for Public Policy Research

further estimated that levelling up health could mean an extra £20 billion gross value added (Thomas et al, 2020).

These opportunity costs are very significant but rarely factored into spatial planning equations. Given the potential cost impacts, why are not all areas planned, designed and built with the underpinning conditions that promote health and wellbeing through a health-promoting environment?

Short-term profits and long-term costs

There are many examples of health-promoting design being delivered across the globe. However, all too often, what is observed is that developers and commissioners from the public or private sector, working within strict financial constraints or timescales, or concerned with meeting specific urgent development needs (such as more housing), will prioritise financial viability or deliverability over meeting other possible social needs.

Planners are sometimes caught in the middle of such dilemmas. This was exemplified in the, now-superseded, 2012 version of the NPPF, which stipulated that the costs of any (local) requirements should 'provide competitive returns to a willing land owner and willing developer to enable the development to be deliverable' (DCLG, 2012: para 173). Other standards and policies – such as seeking health and wellbeing improvements – could not override the need to ensure the financial viability of a project over the economic cycle.

It is noteworthy that this imbalance in viability in favour of the private sector and against the public planning authority was rectified and removed, at least in policy terms, in the most recent iteration of the policy framework (MHCLG, 2019). Although concerns remain that such an imbalance continues to occur in practice, a design guide for England has also been released with 10 features that the UK government believes characterise well-designed places, which it argues should be able to be achieved in practice and will make places 'beautiful, healthy, greener, enduring and successful' (MHCLG, 2021c).

The impact of such guidance has meant that the viability of a project is often measured in quite narrow ways, without taking into account longer-term costs of the project or plans. The longer-term health or wider social costs are rarely factored into the equation of development projects' viability. The consequence is that short-term gains (or profits) are made by (private) developers, with longer-term healthcare and other societal costs falling on the public purse. This is, in effect, a hidden subsidy that the public sector provides to the private or commercial sector, enabling it to build quick and move on, with the public purse picking up the consequences in the longer term.

Physical activity and the urban realm: an example of opportunity lost

> If physical activity were a drug, we would refer to it as a miracle cure, due to the great many illnesses it can prevent and help treat. (UKCMO, 2019)

Physical inactivity is one of the most significant public health challenges facing modern societies, and the evidence to support the health benefits of regular physical activity for all groups is increasingly compelling. Regular physical activity has significant health benefits for individuals. Encouraging physical activity across the population has wider benefits for communities, enabling people to come together to enjoy shared activities when undertaken in a community setting, such as walking, cycling, active recreation, sport and play. It contributes to building strong communities with social, environmental and economic benefits for communities and wider society (UKCMO, 2019; PHE, 2020d).

Designing our towns, communities and neighbourhoods in ways that prioritise active travel and promote physical activity could help reduce the one in six deaths in England that are attributed to lack of physical activity (PHE, 2014). Globally, one in four adults do not meet recommended levels of physical activity, and physically inactive people have a 20 to 30 per cent increased risk of death compared to active people. Up to 5 million deaths a year could be averted if the global population was more active (WHO, 2018b, 2020b).

There is a very strong economic case for taking action now. In England, for example, the estimated cost of physical inactivity is £7.4 billion a year to society and £0.9 billion to the NHS (PHE, 2019a). These economic costs do not include the £5.1 billion costs to society and the NHS arising from poor diet-related ill health (Scarborough et al, 2011), in large part, related to those who are overweight or obese, conditions that are also associated with lack of physical activity.

Challenges and benefits of building and investing in healthy places

This book has summarised the evidence linking the built and natural environment to health and wellbeing, and noted the complex ways in which the environment shapes and influences health and wellbeing. This has underscored the importance of adopting an integrated and holistic HiAP approach to addressing health challenges in spatial planning.

It has shown that although many of the key messages regarding design and health are already known, clear, causal relationships between particular design features and health conditions are difficult to demonstrate. It is even more difficult to demonstrate when making planning decisions in specific locations, as the application of large-scale health and wellbeing studies may – or may not – be directly transferable to what may happen in a development in a specific location.

The challenge for the public health professional is to work with local planners to help interpret such studies and to draw out lessons with general applicability from those that are much more site specific. The other role for the public health professional is to draw out the implications of taking different courses of action on health and wellbeing.

Case study: demonstrating the healthy benefits accruing from a modal shift in transport in the West Midlands, England

The West Midlands Combined Authority (WMCA) is comprised of seven local authorities covering a population of about 3 million people in Central

England. From 2016 to 2021, the WMCA's *Movement for Growth* local transport plan for the development of a transport system for the region was designed to meet the challenges of economic and housing growth, social inclusion, and environment change (WMCA, 2016).

During *Movement for Growth*'s period (2016–21), greater acknowledgement of the challenging health issues that the region's population were now facing was more evident. The transport strategy noted that road transport emissions from exposure to fine particles already accounted for around 1,460 premature deaths in the West Midlands. Therefore, the strategy sought to shift travel modes from cars to more active modes of travel seen in other large European city regions. About 63 per cent of all travel in the West Midlands was made by car, compared to 35 to 45 per cent of all journeys observed in Europe. Due to the wider health-promoting properties of more active lifestyles, it was estimated that shifting to more active modes of travel would result in the following reductions in conditions over a ten-year period:

- 550 fewer cases of type 2 diabetes;
- 1,675 fewer cases of coronary heart disease;
- 625 fewer cases of stroke;
- 125 fewer cases of breast cancer;
- 150 fewer cases of colorectal cancer;
- 3,000 fewer cases of dementia;
- 2,500 fewer cases of depression; and
- 10,000 fewer hip fractures.

The strategy explicitly recognised that when streets are well designed, with health and wellbeing goals in mind, they can be at the heart of cohesive and supportive communities. Streets that make the West Midlands healthier and happier will make the region more economically active, as transport can help increase productivity and reduce the demand for public services by preventing ill health and improving the wellbeing of people at work.

The work has also shown the benefits that can emerge from integrated working between health and transport planners. Embedding a public health professional within the transport department has seen significant refocusing of transport strategies to prioritise health in a number of different authorities.

Note: At the time of writing this, *Movement for Growth* is being replaced by the 'Local transport plan 5 core strategy'.
Source: Transport for West Midlands (2018). Acknowledgement to Duncan Vernon

Benefits of building healthy places

Notwithstanding the short-termism that drives much thinking when it comes to building projects, it is already clear that both consumers and the commercial sector understand, and value, the benefits of well-designed projects that place a premium on health. Developers and volume builders have long understood the value of 'building healthy'; indeed, 'supporting healthy lifestyles' is often used as one of the strong selling points.

Housing development prospectuses for consumers will typically highlight the 'green and leafy' aspects of a development, its 'pleasant surroundings' and 'quiet' streets, and how these support the building of new communities. The UK Office for National Statistics (see Figure 10.1) found that homes within 100 metres of accessible green spaces were on average £2,500 more expensive than if they were more than 500 metres away. This added an average premium to the home of 1.1 per cent. Furthermore, having a view over a green space or water boosted house prices by an extra 1.8 per cent – an average of £4,600.

It should be noted, that this was observed even after allowing for the effects of distance to transport facilities (such as railway stations) and workplaces, and air and noise pollution levels (ONS, 2019). This study was reported before the COVID-19 pandemic, and as observed during the lockdowns and restrictions on movement caused by the pandemic, being close to a green space or park is even more highly prized now among house buyers (ONS, 2021).

The TCPA observed that industry-led benchmarks and standards have increasingly been used by developers and housebuilders as means of accrediting place making and design.

Figure 10.1: Effect of access to green spaces on property prices

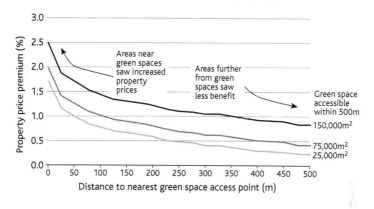

Source: ONS (2019)

Although not necessarily independently verified (though some are), it does demonstrate that the sector recognises the link between profitability and the quality of a housing development (often focusing on resident quality of life and wellbeing benefits) (TCPA, 2018).

Figure 10.2 illustrates the premiums added to the homes and land values of an economy when associated with railway stations, playgrounds, supermarkets, improved pedestrianisation, numbers of street trees or access to a water frontage. For example, it is observed that being located only 500 m rather than 1,500 m from a train station carries a price premium on housing. Is there a similar premium effect on health and wellbeing, or for parks or services? Increasingly, it seems that there is.

Although more difficult to directly measure at such a granular level, the evidence base showing direct health benefits is improving (for example, street trees and mental health) (Marselle et al, 2020). Provision of such amenities as parks and green spaces closer to populations supports people adopting healthier lifestyles and behaviours, with resultant health benefits. In the UK, the 25 Year Environment Plan has set a target to develop standards to ensure that there are high-quality, accessible, natural spaces close to where people live and work, particularly in urban areas, encouraging more people to spend time in them to benefit their health and wellbeing (Defra, 2018; Natural England, 2021).

Figure 10.2: Summary infographic on the value of placemaking elements

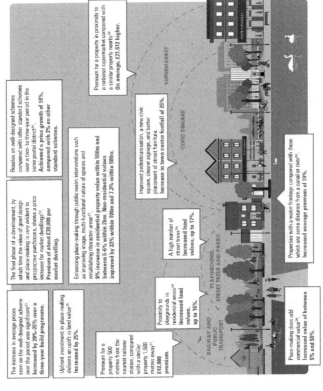

Source: TCPA (2018). For a larger version of this figure, please see: https://www.emcouncils.gov.uk/write/TCPA_-_Securing_Constructive_Collaboration_-_FINAL.pdf

This trend seems to be, if anything, continuing. A study of global real estate investment managers and stakeholders detailed the growth in demand for healthy buildings. The report highlights how in the post-pandemic world of COVID-19, there is increasing investor awareness of the importance of health and wellbeing to their environmental, social and governance (ESG) strategies, as well as the link between building design/function and personal and societal health and wellness. Nearly 90 per cent of those surveyed signalled their intent to enhance their wellness-related asset-management strategies in the coming year.

Investment managers in the study believed that healthy buildings matter: they not only realised rental premiums of between 4.4 and 7.0 per cent, but also observed higher overall productivity, improved employee satisfaction, lower absenteeism and lower turnover. Moving from healthy buildings into neighbourhoods, investment managers themselves recognised how 'walkability' raises home values in US cities (Center for Active Design, 2021).

Balancing trade-offs

It is crucial to be aware of the contrasting outcomes that different stakeholders may hope to realise from a public project. For public health professionals, it is a sobering experience when they realise that their key concerns for a project, for example, seeking better conditions to secure improved health, may be far down the list of priorities that others are hoping to achieve from a plan or project.

Within the 'health' dimension itself, there will generally be multiple, and often competing, priorities (and stakeholders). More health-focused, rapid-assessment checklists, such as the HIAs previously discussed in Chapter 4, look at a range of health-related issues that would be influenced by the built environment. In addition, in order to determine the costs and benefits, individual projects can be assessed by developers or their expert consultants, and 'graded' as to how well they address key issues (see Table 10.1).

In undertaking a cost–benefit assessment, however, different stakeholders will place a different value or priority on achieving such goals in an individual project or within overall planning policies. Key stakeholders might include:

Table 10.1: Planning for healthy places checklist assessment

	Cost–benefit of healthy places			
Parameters	Positive	Negative	Neutral	Uncertain
Housing quality and design				
Access to healthcare services and other social infrastructure				
Access to open space and nature				
Air quality, noise and neighbourhood amenity				
Accessiblity and active transport				
Crime reduction and community safety				
Access to healthy food				
Access to work and training				
Social cohesion and lifetime neighbourhoods				
Minimising the use of resources				
Climate change				
Health inequalities				

Source: Adapted from Nottinghamshire County Council (2019)

Public and voluntary sector:

- individuals, local and neighbouring communities, community organisations, and regional and national interested parties;
- spatial planners;
- public health teams; and
- decision-makers, that is, planning committees/elected officials (politicians).

Private sector:

- commercial sector, for example, for goods and services;
- architects, engineers, builders, developers and commissioned consultants; and
- financiers, investors and landowners.

Balancing competing priorities across these groups is difficult; the challenge is to identify and articulate how benefits can be realised in ways that maximise the win–wins for all. Use of tools such as HIA or benchmarks and standards (preferably those that are independently verified) will help to bridge, or at least identify, gaps. Decisions also need to be taken within the context of current national policy guidance.

Understanding the tools at the disposal of different sectors and the impacts on health and wellbeing can help. For public health professionals, supporting those in the planning and building sectors to understand the impact of their designs, plans and projects on health and wellbeing is part of this. On the other hand, understanding the processes, underpinning finances, timescales and risks facing these sectors by public health and other decision-makers will enable public health professionals to engage more effectively and add value to the process (TCPA, 2018).

Balancing competing priorities is difficult. However, when the government's design guidance, as now established in England (MHCLG, 2021c), have 'health' peppered throughout as an integral theme showing a clear understanding of the impacts that the built environment can have, much of the groundwork has already been laid for public health professionals.

Low-traffic neighbourhoods: a case study in trade-offs

The health benefits of more pedestrian-friendly neighbourhoods have been increasingly recognised in policymaking and project development. In one Vancouver study, it was found that people living in pedestrian-friendly neighbourhoods walked three times more a week for transportation than those living in car-dependent areas and were found to have a lower incidence of high blood pressure and rates of obesity (Frank et al, 2014). The 'walkability premium' for both domestic and commercial premises has already been noted by investment managers (Center for Active Design, 2021).

In many towns and cities in the UK and elsewhere, there are proposals for the development of low-traffic neighbourhoods (LTNs). LTNs have been defined as 'a scheme where motor vehicle traffic in residential streets is greatly reduced. This is done by minimising the amount of traffic that comes from vehicles using the streets to get to another destination (often referred to as "through-traffic" or "rat-running")' (Sustrans, 2021).

LTNs are designed to enhance the local environment by reducing the volume of traffic and thereby reducing collisions, improving air quality, reducing noise and, specifically, prioritising local residents so that they can better enjoy their local neighbourhood. More generally, they seek to enhance local community life by reducing road traffic on local roads. These are, of course, all things that go to support the conditions for better health and wellbeing.

LTNs are often 'sold' by supporters as opening up networks of streets so local people can safely travel through the area on foot, bicycles and other wheeled transport, as well as public transport, and still allow private motorised vehicles to have easy access to homes and businesses. Although majority views are supportive, in practice, these have often been extremely controversial to implement, with opposition coming not just from the road lobby and locals onto whose roads the traffic is redirected, but often from the local commercial sector, which sometimes views this as likely to have a negative impact on business (Aldred and Verlinghieri, 2020; Griffiths, 2021).

The impact of LTNs on people living with disabilities, and the future of accessible active travel

In its *Pave the Way* report about LTNs, Transport for All (2021) concluded that participants reported easier or more pleasant journeys, an increase in independence, a decrease in traffic danger, and benefits to physical and mental health. Criticisms included longer journey times for residents, as well as for their visitors who provide care and support. This leads to travel becoming more exhausting, expensive, complicated and difficult. There were also cases of a negative impact on mental health, issues with taxis and a perceived rise in traffic danger.

However, with many people living with disabilities experiencing genuine and meaningful benefits from LTNs, ripping them out and returning to normal is not the solution. 'Normal' – what we had before – was not accessible enough either. The answer involves engaging with and listening to the perspectives of people living with disabilities, who have been significantly erased from the conversation. Only then can accessible and inclusive solutions be found that benefit everyone and the environment.

Gentrification: an example of health inequalities

Redevelopment of urban neighbourhoods carries its own challenges with regard to gentrification. Although people know what gentrification is when they see it, to define it and measure the impacts that gentrification has on health and wellbeing has been a challenge for researchers. There is also evidence that investment managers have increasingly come to recognise how 'healthy buildings' equal 'healthy balance sheets'. But what are the impacts of wholesale neighbourhood improvements on health and community wellbeing more generally? Are there 'right' and 'wrong' ways to improve local environments so as to guarantee improvements in health for everyone?

Gentrification has generally been defined as the process whereby a neighbourhood becomes upwardly mobile through an influx of individuals, often younger urban professionals, who have a higher socio-economic status than the existing population. Gentrification can result in improved housing for individuals and an improved physical environment in the neighbourhood. However, it can also: increase prices for housing, goods and services; displace the existing population; change the racial composition of the neighbourhood; and have a range of impacts on social networks, crime and, as some research literature is beginning to demonstrate, health and wellbeing.

A systematic review by Bhavsar et al (2020) observed that the impact of gentrification on health was not uniform across populations, with marginalised populations, such as black residents and older people, impacted more than white and younger residents. A range of psychosocial and physical effects were observed in the different studies, though one possible mechanism postulated by which gentrification impacts on health is through the disruption to social capital that previously held the community together. Bhavsar et al (2020) developed a model

Figure 10.3: Model of gentrification, changes to the environment and health outcomes

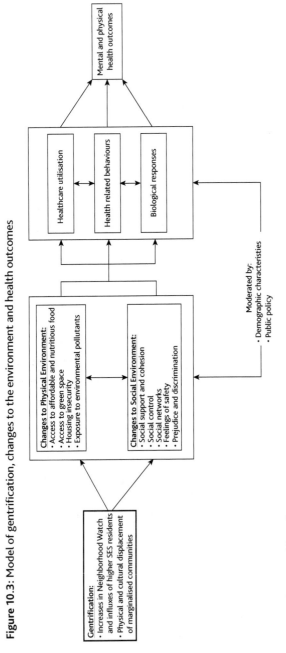

Source: Bhavsar et al (2020)

demonstrating how the interplay between changes to the built environment and the social environment could have a range of effects on health-related behaviour, healthcare-related behaviour and biological responses, such as stress, leading to differential physical and mental health outcomes (see Figure 10.3). Developing consensus and achieving equitable outcomes for all sectors in such circumstances is a delicate balancing act, requiring the engagement of all stakeholders – not least the local community involved. Gentrification illustrates the nature of the interactions between the built environment and the social environment, and how these will, in turn, influence health and wellbeing. When overlaid with a range of stakeholders, each with different priorities or seeking different outcomes to varying timescales, this makes consensus difficult. Holding the line to ensure that there are health and wellbeing improvements for all as a result of the development can be more challenging still.

Points of intervention for health

This chapter has explored some of the competing challenges facing public health professionals and planners when attempting to plan for healthy new communities or when redeveloping older ones. However, a more challenging ask is to make the case and achieve consensus on how to create a healthy, viable place.

Some reviews have identified the attributes, skills and other components, such as promoting good governance, that are required to have any hope of developing sustainable communities through the planning system (Egan Review, 2004). Recently, with respect to housing, key pinch points in the planning process have been mapped (see Figure 10.4), showing those critical stages when interventions to deliver design value can be made (White et al, 2020).

From a public health perspective, it is important that practitioners understand the local process and agree on those specific stages in which they can have maximum impact on the development of policies or specific projects. For their part, local health stakeholders need to set out a clear statement of the specific health challenges facing their communities to ensure that wider discussions on community needs for infrastructure,

Figure 10.4: Critical points of interventions to maximise value from design

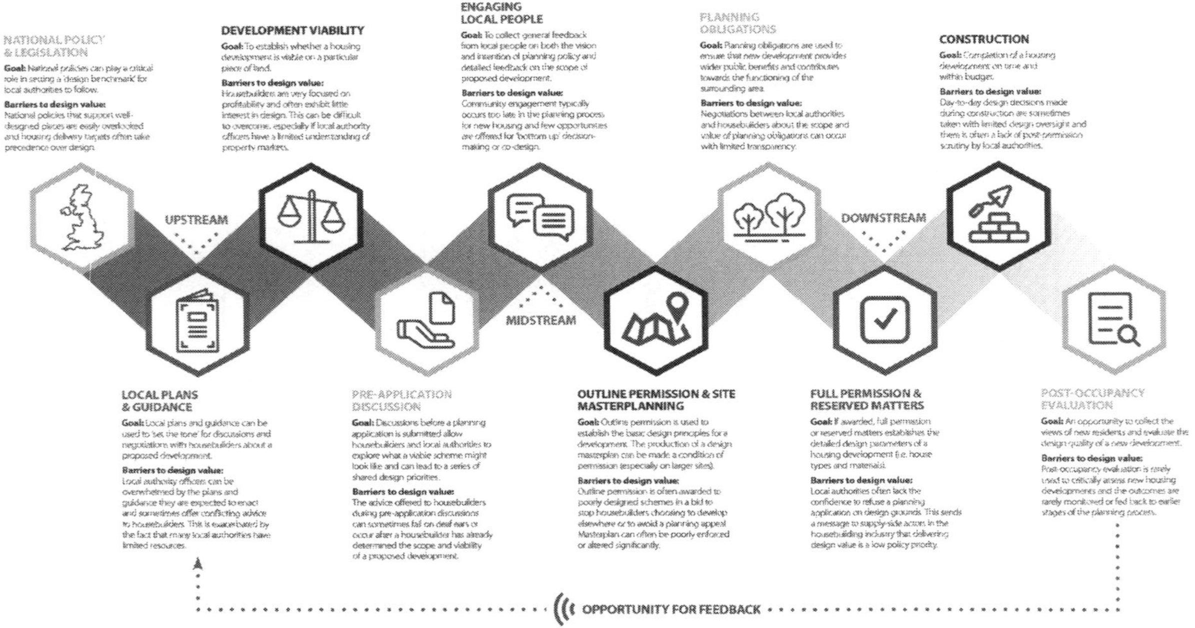

NATIONAL POLICY & LEGISLATION

Goal: National policies can play a critical role in setting a design benchmark for local authorities to follow.

Barriers to design value: National policies that support well-designed places are easily overlooked, and housing delivery targets often take precedence over design.

DEVELOPMENT VIABILITY

Goal: To establish whether a housing development is viable on a particular piece of land.

Barriers to design value: Housebuilders are very focused on profitability and often exploit little interest in design. This can be difficult to overcome, especially if local authority officers have a limited understanding of property markets.

ENGAGING LOCAL PEOPLE

Goal: To collect general feedback from local people on both the vision and intention of planning policy and detailed feedback on the scope of proposed development.

Barriers to design value: Community engagement typically occurs too late in the planning process for new housing, and few opportunities are offered for bottom-up decision-making or co-design.

PLANNING OBLIGATIONS

Goal: Planning obligations are used to ensure that new development provides wider public benefits and contributes towards the functioning of the surrounding area.

Barriers to design value: Negotiations between local authorities and housebuilders about the scope and value of planning obligations can occur with limited transparency.

CONSTRUCTION

Goal: Completion of a housing development on time and within budget.

Barriers to design value: Day-to-day design decisions made during construction are sometimes taken with limited design oversight and then is often a lack of post permission scrutiny by local authorities.

POST-OCCUPANCY EVALUATION

Goal: An opportunity to collect the views of new residents and evaluate the design quality of a new development.

Barriers to design value: Post-occupancy evaluation is rarely used to critically assess how housing developments and the outcomes are rarely monitored or fed back to earlier stages of the planning process.

LOCAL PLANS & GUIDANCE

Goal: Local plans and guidance can be used to set the tone for discussions and negotiations with housebuilders about a proposed development.

Barriers to design value: Local authority officers can be overwhelmed by the plans and guidance they are expected to enact and sometimes offer conflicting advice to housebuilders. This is exacerbated by the fact that many local authorities have limited resources.

PRE-APPLICATION DISCUSSION

Goal: Discussions before a planning application is submitted allow housebuilders and local authorities to explore what a viable scheme might look like and can lead to a series of shared design priorities.

Barriers to design value: The advice offered to housebuilders during pre-application discussions can sometimes fall too deaf ears or occur after a housebuilder has already determined the scope and viability of a proposed development.

OUTLINE PERMISSION & SITE MASTERPLANNING

Goal: Outline permission is used to establish the basic design principles for a development. The production of a design masterplan can be made a condition of permission (especially on larger sites).

Barriers to design value: Outline permission is often awarded to poorly designed schemes in a bid to stop housebuilders choosing to develop elsewhere or to avoid a planning appeal. Masterplans can often be poorly enforced or allowed significantly.

FULL PERMISSION & RESERVED MATTERS

Goal: If awarded, full permission or reserved matters establishes the detailed design parameters of a housing development (i.e. house types and materials).

Barriers to design value: Local authorities often lack the confidence to refuse a planning application on design grounds. This sends a message to supply-side actors in the housebuilding industry that delivering design value is a low policy priority.

UPSTREAM

MIDSTREAM

DOWNSTREAM

(((OPPORTUNITY FOR FEEDBACK

Source: White et al (2020: xxiii). Reproduced with the kind permission of the UK Collaborative Centre for Housing Evidence, funded by the Economic and Social Research Council, the Arts and Humanities Research Council and the Joseph Rowntree Foundation. For a larger version of this figure, please see: https://housingevidence.ac.uk/wp-content/uploads/2020/12/Delivering_design_value_critical_points_of_intervention.jpg

housing and green spaces, for example, are informed by such assessments (Department of Health, 2011).

Developing a local health and planning agenda

A local initiative that systematically attempts to develop a local health and planning agenda would go a long way to ensuring that healthy, sustainable developments can be secured for the community. Such a local programme needs to ensure that:

- health professionals identify the demographic and health challenges facing the local community, and how these can best be addressed in local spatial plans and developments as part of wider health strategies seeking health and wellbeing improvements;
- national and local design policies focusing on health and wellbeing are developed to guide developers, so that health impacts are identified and cost–benefit analyses are integrated into projects from the start;
- governance arrangements are in place that enable stakeholders to be identified, relationships built and outcomes and aims of projects clarified from the beginning in order to ensure that lasting health value and outcomes can result from the project;
- all stakeholders – especially the local community – are involved in clarifying the aims, objectives and outcomes of the project, supported by evidence and clarity as to how these will be monitored and evaluated, and agree what success looks like in health terms in the short and longer term; and
- due consideration is given to possible unintended consequences, for example, the implications that a redesigned built environment can have on the wider social environment, how this may impact on health and wellbeing outcomes, and how project design can address any unintended consequences.

Concluding statement

The messages seem clear: in any planning project, there is a balance to be struck between benefits, costs and the trade-offs that are necessary to be made between stakeholders with different aims, objectives and agendas. There is a good body of evidence to show the opportunities for better health and wellbeing that can be achieved if 'health' considerations are prioritised from the start of the project. Indeed, if they are not, there is a danger of significant health impacts and healthcare costs being stored up for the future.

To ensure that health needs are addressed in local plans and projects, it is essential that there is good communication between built environment and health professionals, as well as others engaged in the planning process. By addressing and engaging with the concerns of the local community, and by ensuring that local health needs are incorporated into all stages of the design and planning of infrastructure projects, policymakers, planners and built environment and public health professionals will be able to support the development of sustainable and healthy places.

11

Securing value

There are many other important intangibles which
contribute to value. Because markets do not trade
explicitly in these things, it is hard to identify and
quantify their value. Intangible factors in health,
happiness and wellbeing, for example, have the
potential to keep the cost of health services affordable
and are only now becoming better recognised.

RICS (2016, p 45)

A function of public health spatial planning practice is to help
identify and secure value from development to achieve health
outcomes. The objective of procuring evidence to support healthy
policy creation and decisions on planning applications is being
able to identify value from development. This will allow public
authorities to secure tangible contributions from developers and
those who finance and build developments to support healthy
place creation (Chang, 2017). These contributions include
providing a range of items alongside residential units, including
affordable housing, community infrastructure and open spaces,
the health benefits of which were set out in Chapter 10. When
such contributions, which can be a significant sum of money, are
allocated and spent appropriately, they can make a meaningful
impact on the health and wellbeing of the community.

This chapter describes the principles and process of planning
gain to secure the necessary financial and system investment in
elements that promote health. It will highlight the planning

mechanisms for financial contributions, with examples of where local authorities have helped secured contributions for health benefit. This chapter highlights:

- using planning to secure developer contributions for health;
- the scale of financial developer contributions; and
- developer contributions and inequalities in places.

Using planning to secure contributions for health

It has been a long-standing principle and ethical position that planning permissions cannot be bought. This means that gaining consent should not be dependent on whether and how much community value and benefits (financial or otherwise) will accrue from the development. This does not mean that values and benefits cannot be a material consideration or necessarily detached from the decision-making process. Indeed, a system of developer contributions exists in most planning systems to financially mitigate against development impact and/or help harness the rise in land values associated with development for community benefit.

Development contributions

Development contributions are a mechanism through which the local authority is able to secure a combination of financial, non-financial and in-kind contributions for planning purposes as a condition for granting planning consent. They are often used to mitigate adverse impacts, as well as to invest in the local infrastructure and services necessary to address additional pressures from new development. They can also be known across different systems as 'planning obligations', 'planning agreements', 'financial contributions' or 'planning gain'.

It is also important to recognise who pays and who benefits in planning, and where the power and responsibilities lie. Chapter 10 identified the multiple beneficiaries of the benefits of planning for health, which provides a sound and fair basis for determining who should contribute and by how much. A good starting position is to adopt the well-known sustainable development principle that the 'polluter pays', first set out in the 1992 Rio Declaration, in which the polluter will seek to internalise the environmental impact costs for public benefit (United Nations, 1992).

For example, if a development with commercial or industrial activities will result in identifiable harm to people's wellbeing from excessive noise pollution and the planning applicant cannot prevent and avoid this harm, they should be expected to make a contribution to mitigate and reduce the impact, such as installing double-glazed windows or noise barriers. Tangible harms, such as noise and air pollution and, most recently, carbon emissions, can be readily identified and addressed to minimise impact to acceptable quantifiable levels, and the polluter pays principle has been effectively applied in such contexts. In addition, the approach is being applied in a developing context to biodiversity offsetting in order to compensate for measurable biodiversity loses as a result of development (Defra, 2012).

Net health gain

Planning for health will often address intangible issues of improved wellbeing at both individual and population levels, such as actions to reduce social isolation and protect mental health, which can make it more challenging to quantify what contributions will be needed (RICS, 2016). The concept of 'net health gain' is being explored in the context of improving outdoor air quality (PHE, 2019b). This means that proposed urban development should deliver an overall measurable benefit to people's health and wellbeing (for an example of the air-quality intervention hierarchy, see Figure 11.1), which, in effect, means that any new development should be healthy by design.

Such consideration to deliver net gains to health will keep developers incentivised so that design and investment strategies clearly set out a tangible approach to prevent and mitigate against ill health, and then maintain and promote good health and wellbeing. Planning at the local level should be about achieving a

Figure 11.1: Net health gain and intervention hierarchy

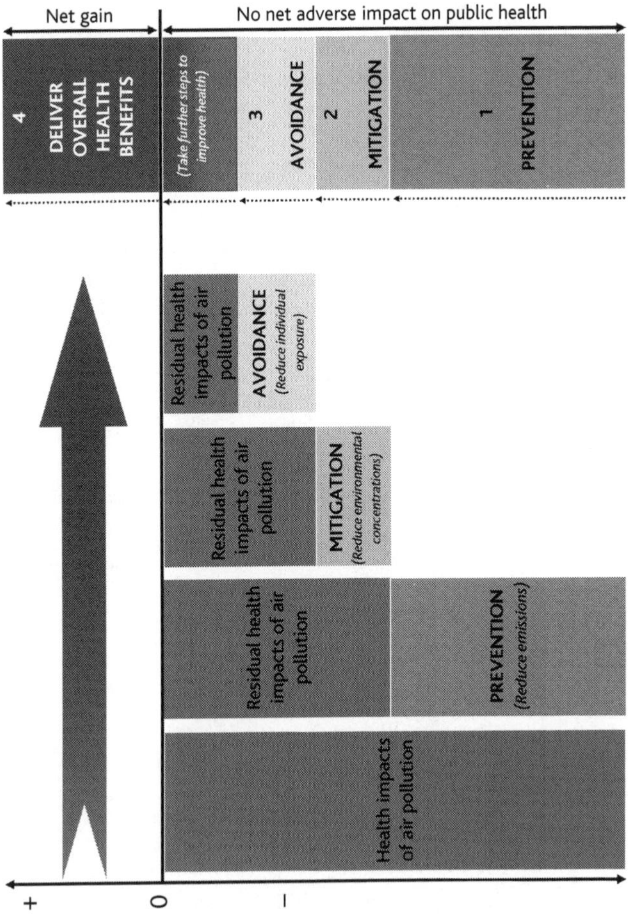

'net health gain', using local health and care needs as the baseline, implemented in collaboration with public health practitioners.

Types of contributions

The planning system has various levers to identify and help secure contributions as part of the development process in order both to prevent and protect against harms and to promote health gains. These contributions are secured from planning applicants as part of the process of applying for consent and will relate to the type and scale of proposed development. They can be financial, non-financial or in-kind.

Types of contributions from development

- Financial: monetary payment direct to the public authority or a specified beneficiary to build or deliver a service or programme, or employ specialist posts, such as a travel planner.
- Non-financial: non-monetised contribution that can include a requirement to undertake an action, such as an assessment, or to prevent actions being undertaken.
- In-kind: the applicant is required to undertake a specified action directly or indirectly, such as building a cycle lane, playground or a structure.

Tests for securing contributions

Applicants can range from the average person wanting to build an extension to their home, to the major corporate house builder creating a new neighbourhood. It is important to be transparent about the reason for contributions. There are conditions or tests as to what and how contributions should be secured. These can be set out in legislation or policy (Scottish Government, 2020; MHCLG, 2019), and refined through case law and established practice.

Four tests (see Table 11.1) determine that a decision be made to secure contributions for health when it:

Table 11.1: Use of developer contributions for planning for health purposes assessed against the four tests

Proposed contributions	Test 1: Necessary	Test 2: Purpose	Test 3: Planning related	Test 4: Reasonable
Public realm improvements, such as seating to increase accessibility in the area	✓	✓	✓	✓
Commission an HIA for a house extension prior to development commencing and being approved by the public authority	X	✓	✓	X
Commission an HIA for a new neighbourhood prior to development commencing and being approved by the public authority	X	✓	✓	✓
Support a local weight-management programme in the proposed development area with high obesity levels	X	X	X	X
Provide a local youth centre for a new neighbourhood to allow communities to hold training and other events	✓	✓	✓	✓
Make a financial contribution for upgrading a local hospital due to projected increased demand from new housing	✓	✓	✓	✓

- is *necessary* to make the proposed development acceptable in planning terms, with part of the consideration for this test being whether the contribution could be better secured through other means;
- serves a *planning purpose* and relates to development plans, as the contribution should be related to the purpose of planning that is about the use and development of land, and to achieve requirements set out in plans and policies;
- *relates* to the proposed development, which means that the requirement for a contribution should be as a direct consequence of the development or arising from the cumulative impact of development in the area; and
- is *reasonable* in scale and kind to the proposed development.

Types of contributions

Public authorities will usually set out their requirements in policy or guidance documents on how much contribution will be required and the eligible items on which contributions can be spent. To support more specific contributions for health, there is the opportunity to cross-check against the planning for health checklists in planning policy on the elements that make up healthy places to determine the type and quantity of contributions needed.

Table 11.2 highlights some examples of general types of contributions set out by public authorities that can contribute towards planning for health, according to the key themes highlighted in Chapter 1 based on evidence. This list is not exhaustive, and the options will depend on meeting the four tests and local circumstances.

Contributions relating to procedural costs

Fees payable to the public authority to obtain consent are separate to the issues of contributions. They are used to maintain the planning department's level of corporate service, such as technical and administrative staff time to process applications, review associated documents and undertake public consultations. Such

Table 11.2: Examples of items eligible for developer contributions that can be used for planning for health purposes

Themes	Examples of items
Neighbourhood design	• Children's play spaces • Healthy development and design certification • Sports grounds and playing fields • Street lighting, furniture and signage
Housing	• Temporary housing to address homelessness • Specialist housing for people with learning disabilities or wheelchair users • Meeting sustainable and energy-efficient home standards
Food environment	• Healthy catering commitments and certification • Food-growing spaces and allotments
Natural environment	• Planting of new street trees and other greening and public realm improvement initiatives • Flood risk management measures and buffers to homes
Transport	• New pedestrian crossings • Air-quality mitigation measures or financial contributions • Travel planner post and annual monitoring and reporting • Shared car clubs
Healthcare and social infrastructure	• Early years and childcare education facilities or financial contributions based on new homes and student numbers • Community, primary and acute healthcare facility or integrated health hubs

fees can be set nationally or locally. For example, in England, planning fees are set nationally and can range from £96 for a large home extension to a maximum of £300,000 for a significant housing development.

Application fees are relevant to discussions in planning for health. This is because fees correspond to the level of service public authorities are able to resource, particularly in periods of reduced public administration grants, and consequently to their ability and capacity to engage with public health teams proactively. This issue is particularly acute in systems without a strong legislative or policy basis for planning for health. In part, this explains the importance of the role of public health spatial planning practitioner in Chapter 9 to introduce and maintain both capability and capacity in public authorities.

Scale of development contributions

The planning system secures a significant amount of financial contributions to public authorities and local communities through the planning applications process. Contributions are secured as a condition of consent for development and as part of a negotiation process with planning applicants, landowners or developers. It is important to understand that these contributions are needed to:

- prevent, reduce or mitigate impact from the specified development, which continues to be the primary directive for securing contributions;
- meet identified shortfalls or funding gaps for infrastructure and services needs arising from population growth/changes from new development; and
- meet additional investment needs as part of a wider planning and infrastructure strategy associated with expected population growth/changes.

Total amount of developer contributions and eligible items

The scale of the contributions from development secured through the planning system annually should not be understated. Development models have evolved to include contributions alongside other development costs as part of the overall viability assessment of a scheme. In an economy where priorities are focused on maximising economic potential from growth and development, contributions generated by the planning process can be an important source of investment in direct or indirect health-promoting interventions.

In England, government-commissioned studies estimated the total value of contributions and for what items these contributions were provided. The total amount collected in one year in 2018–19 was nearly £7 billion by those local authorities with planning functions in England. This was an

Table 11.3: Estimated value of developer contributions in England, Wales and Scotland

England	Wales	Scotland
Total = £6.9 billion (2018–19)	Total = £28.8 million (2005–06)	Total = £490 million (2019–20)
Affordable housing £4.675 billion	Affordable housing £16.8 million	Affordable housing £310 million
Open space and environment £157 million	Open space and environment £4.2 million	Other infrastructure (Education, transport, open/green space, sporting and recreational, medical facilities/ emergency services) £180 million
Transport and travel £294 million	Transport and travel £2.8 million	
Education £439 million	Education £1.5 million	
Community works £62 million	Community works £839,000	

Source: For England, Lord et al (2020); for Wales, Rowley et al (2007); and for Scotland, Blanc et al (2021)

increase of 17 per cent from the total of £5.7 billion collected in 2006–07. These studies show that the contributions fund the provision of several items, including a majority and increasing proportion of both affordable housing and education facilities, though decreasing proportion of both transport and open spaces. Table 11.3 presents the value of contributions for three UK nations that use similar methodologies, though different time periods, according to the latest available published studies.

Comparisons to public health services

The total receipt of developer contributions can be comparable to budgets from other functions, such as the public health department. For example, the £6.9 billion in contributions secured in one year by local authorities in England from development is nearly double the budget allocated to local authority public health departments (see the following box). Local authorities will retain the receipts from contributions and spend them according to local infrastructure needs and priorities, often set out in a local infrastructure list. This offers the opportunity for additional levels of investment in health-promoting interventions to support public health priorities around planning for health. However, determining where and what appropriate interventions could be supported by developer contributions will require explicit engagement from the planning and public health departments, in accordance with the four tests set out earlier.

Comparison of the scale of developer contributions to the public health budget in England

A total of £7 billion was secured from developer contributions in England in one year in 2018–19. To gain a sense of scale, £3.324 billion overall was provided from public health ring-fenced grants to the 152 local authorities with public health functions in England for 2021–22 (DHSC, 2021). This grant can be used by the local directors of public health for both revenue and capital expenditure for a range of functions to fulfil their statutory public health responsibilities.

Resourcing and skills

Agreeing contributions to provide items is only the start of the process, and local authorities need to be able to secure timely receipt and then invest and spend the money in ways that meet their identified local infrastructure needs. In practice, a large amount of the contributions lie unspent, with one investigation finding local authorities only spending 37 per cent of contributions received from developers (Lanktree, 2019) and developers experiencing delays in agreeing contributions during the planning application process.

Local authorities have faced consistent challenges around capacity, with few having dedicated officers to manage contributions and the skills to effectively negotiate with developers (Crook et al, 2006). Many of the local authorities with smaller planning teams or in areas of relative stability in terms of planning activity may not have the need or the access to capability that other areas experiencing growth or larger metropolitan areas will have.

Knowledge of development economics has been identified as an essential skill for planners (Adams, 2021). Good working knowledge of development economics allows planners to engage with interested stakeholders (including those working in the health sector) in order to secure the necessary policy objectives or infrastructure, while these stakeholders also need a reciprocal understanding of development economics (Roger Tym & Partners, 2010). Without the necessary knowledge, it is challenging for public health teams to have the kind of meaningful engagement with planners to make the case for and allocate contributions towards appropriate health-promoting interventions. This is a role that a public health spatial planning practitioner can help fill.

Developer contributions and inequalities in places

While the overall scale of contributions secured can be significant, their distribution will vary from area to area. Understanding the relationship between the scale and level of contributions and inequalities is dependent on the following factors:

- Housing market and demand: areas with higher growth and demand will result in applications for more and larger developments, which will translate into increased contributions secured from these developments.
- Land values: values attributed to the site by the developer as part of viability calculations represent the parameters within which to assess the affordable level of contributions, including profit allowances (RICS, 2012).
- Resourcing and skills: the ability of local authorities to secure contributions is influenced by having the necessary skills and knowledge of practitioners, as well as the strength of policy and processes (Rowley et al, 2007).

When breaking down the overall contributions figure of £6.9 billion by English regions, a pattern of spatial inequalities begins to become visible (see Figure 11.2). Areas that experience high housing growth and property demand in the south of England are able to secure higher levels of developer contributions,

Figure 11.2: Regional breakdown of developer contributions for 2018–19 in England

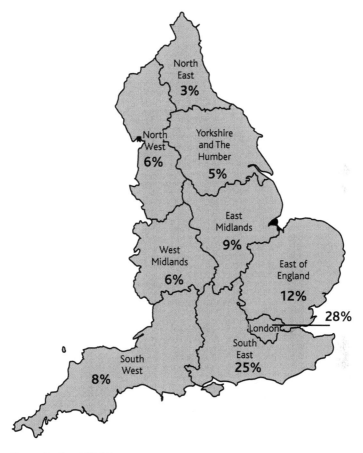

Source: Lord et al (2020)

which can, in turn, be used to invest in a higher quality of environment. However, in areas that experience lower levels of housing growth and demand, such as in the north of England, the prospect of securing meaningful levels of developer contributions is diminished due to viability concerns. Furthermore, there are areas with constrained geographies, in which there are predominantly smaller-scale developments that are exempt from making contributions or too small to make a significant contribution, despite having cumulative impacts that can be just as significant as a single development.

When placing contributions, for example, by regional breakdown, against people's lifestyles, public service provision and health outcomes, patterns begin to emerge. Can public authorities better repurpose the use of developer contributions to help reduce health inequalities by investing in the infrastructure items that specific areas need? For example, in transport, the share of adults cycling at least five times per week and the share of adults walking at least five times per week were lowest in parts of the north of England, such as in Burnley (0.1 per cent) and Middlesbrough (21 per cent), respectively (Health Foundation, 2021). Can developer contributions be more fairly used to invest in active travel interventions to improve physical activity and ultimately close the healthy life expectancy gap existing in many places?

In another example, regional variations were also found in housing quality by a design audit of 142 housing developments across England based on categories of design considerations, such as environment and community, streets, and parking and pedestrian experience (Place Alliance, 2020). Schemes assessed from the north-east, north-west and south-west of England scored below the English average, with mediocre and poor scores. Can developer contributions and stronger planning policy decisions help secure better housing quality?

Further breaking down the figures to neighbourhoods within a local authority can help understand why inequalities continue to exist in society. The most desirable places will have higher land values and therefore attract higher and continual demand for development, while the least desirable places, though in need of improvement, will not attract investment due to suppressed demand. These least desirable places have a set of complex socio-economic challenges and historic underinvestment, which have contributed to the neglect of the physical environment. However, these are also the areas with the greatest need for investment. With the quality of new developments depending on the value of land, planners and those working in public authorities feel that they have been unable to deliver on many planning-related public policy objectives, including healthy place making (APSE, 2020).

In some circumstances, regulatory interventions in planning in the context of a market-led property economy can contribute to the unintended institutionalisation of inequalities. For example, English local authorities are able to introduce a community infrastructure levy (CIL), a form of development tax, in addition to what is known as Section 106 developer contributions. However, due to viability assessments that would make any development in areas of low land values unviable, these areas (often regeneration areas) are exempt from CIL. If left unchecked by changes making regulation, policy interventions and investment decisions fairer, this pattern of unintended institutionalised inequalities can further exacerbate the levels of health inequalities visible today.

Local authorities set appropriate thresholds for developer contributions in order to provide clarity as to when contributions will be sought. In setting thresholds, the public authority intends to balance the objective of ensuring that new development makes a proportionate contribution to the requirements it will generate, with the objective of not overburdening smaller developments and businesses that do not typically generate the economies of scale and impact that larger developments and corporations do.

Social value in planning for health

Social value is understood as the extent to which activities and built places improve economic, social and environmental wellbeing, and provide benefits to local communities (UKGBC, 2020; Urban Land Institute, 2021). There is an increasing interest shown in developing social value considerations in the planning and development process.

Public sector bodies in the UK are already subject to social value duties under the Public Services (Social Value) Act 2012 but private sector bodies are voluntarily adopting a similar approach. The Urban Land Institute's (2021) surveys in Europe and globally found that private sector actors in real estate also have a strong interest in social value creation in relation to their corporate social responsibility or ESG functions. This chimes with the strengthening evidence in Chapter 10 on the financial value of healthy and quality places and environments recognised by developers, landowners and investors.

In planning, many of the planning mechanisms highlighted, such as developer contributions, local plans and planning decision-making, can be used to set social value requirements. In a market-led economy, where planning is largely driven by private sector developers, making the case for social value and setting out clear social value policy as part of planning for health can mean a win–win for everyone.

Concluding statement

The planning and development process secures a significant amount of contributions and value added to public and private sector actors, including local authorities and developers. If unchecked in a market-led property economy and market-driven planning process, there is a danger of exacerbating what is already an indirect form of institutionalised inequalities built into the value system in planning. Public health spatial planning practice can harness the scale of contributions to reorient local investment to health-promoting interventions and rebalance where these interventions can be put in place to reduce health inequalities.

Insider story 11.1: Using voluntary building standards in delivering health and wellbeing

Harry Knibb, a real estate development professional, and Olga Turner Baker, co-founder of health and wellbeing design consultancy Ekkist, highlight their experiences and lessons learned from the early days of voluntary healthy building certifications through a UK project case study.

The role of wildlife trusts as delivery partners for health, wellbeing and social value in spatial planning

Wildlife trusts in the UK own and manage over 2,300 nature reserves, covering 98,500 hectares, and operate more than 100 visitor and education centres. Given this scale, reach and inherent alignment, wildlife trusts have a large role to play in the delivery of public health and wellbeing, as well as social value, within the UK's overall spatial planning strategy.

In 2017, Kent Wildlife Trust ran an international design competition for a nature and wellbeing centre, with the goal of creating 'the first centre of its kind in the country dedicated to connecting people and nature in ways that evidence and demonstrate positive benefits for both people and wildlife'. The aim of the project was to: raise awareness of the importance of conservation work for people's health and wellbeing, as well as that of the planet; encourage a wider range of visitors, such as those from the nearby housing estates, alongside the existing nature enthusiasts, ornithologists and anglers; and engage with wider-scale initiatives, such as the NHS social prescribing framework.

The competition was won by a project team led by architects Studio McLeod and Ekkist, alongside nine other professional disciplines, highlighting the need for a joined-up approach in addressing the many aspects of design, sustainability, planning and wellbeing required to deliver a comprehensive masterplan and building design. The team's approach was to create 'symbiosis' between nature, people and architecture, where nature supports human wellbeing and people are, in turn, more motivated to support the wellbeing of nature. This built on the site's pioneering history as the first industrial gravel pit redeveloped for wildlife and conservation, with a further aim of becoming the first visitor centre in the world to achieve WELL Building Standard™ certification, using this as a driver for both social and commercial value to the project.

Execution

The design response was focused on simple, natural building materials that were not only low cost to construct, but also had aesthetic elements that reflected the 'wilding' nature of the site. Belfast 'lattice' trusses were designed as both a cost-effective solution that reflected biophilic design and to directly reference bird wings and nests. A daylight-first approach was taken to lighting the building, as well as an electric lighting strategy that minimised its impact on wildlife and simultaneously supported occupants' circadian rhythms. Timber interiors were inspired by birdwatching hides and the Kent vernacular, as well as their calming properties and indoor air-quality benefits. Rammed-earth walls referenced early Kent ragstone buildings and the gravel quarry, while hempcrete insulated the walls and provided a breathable membrane. Mental health and wellbeing were also considered by following detailed design guidance for autism, Asperger's syndrome and a range of mental health issues in order to ensure inclusivity for a wider range of user groups.

The layout was organised so that the noisy, quiet and private functions of reception and cafe, exhibition and studio, and treatment rooms, respectively, could coexist without disruption, and provided spaces for refuge and seclusion, as well as considering the interaction with wildlife, so that nature could thrive alongside growing visitor numbers harmoniously. Constraints included such factors as a client who had recently not been involved with the planning and development process, a highly environmentally sensitive site and a phased budget that was to be released in stages dependent on fundraising activities.

Outcome

The projected budget of the competition scheme and review of the overall strategy, including net zero carbon, resulted in an alternative scaled-back approach, where the existing centre would be refurbished and extended instead. WELL Building Standard™ certification was not a consideration for the new brief; however, the core principles of healthy and sustainable building design remained, including the benefits of social prescribing already provided by the reserve. A full project team, which included a local architect, was appointed to execute the refurbishment and extension of the existing centre and the wider works required on the reserve, including rationalised car parking.

Despite this, the key message and overall principles remained, including the delivery of a high-quality place that allows people to engage more with nature, attracts a wider target audience and builds on the site's ability to generate social value for the local community. The planning response was positive due to the synergies with the NPPF and with sustainability, health and wellbeing goals.

Observable lessons: early adopter or late follower?

The observable lessons from industry experience and this case study have shown there to be both economic and social motivations for design for wellbeing and the use of voluntary health and wellbeing building certifications. There is a clear distinction emerging between 'early adopters' (such as those outlined in the case study) and those who are now concerned with being 'late followers' and playing catch-up, albeit within a voluntary regulation framework.

While economic motivations are often concerned with product differentiation and value premiums, social motivations are often aligned with companies' wider social and ESG frameworks, and social responsibility and transparency initiatives. There is clearly a shift happening from 'being first' to 'not being the last' to adopt these standards, which focus on accountability, transparency and, ultimately, the developers' and investors' responsibility through the buildings constructed and masterplans drawn.

Further information

Further details of the Wildlife Trusts project case study are available at: www.architecture.com/awards-and-competitions-landing-page/competitions-landing-page/sevenoaks-nature-and-wellbeing-centre

Insider story 11.2: Developers' commitment to a healthy development in Acton Gardens, London, England

Andrew Taylor, Group Planning Director for Countryside Partnerships, highlights the role of developers in securing healthy developments through a project case study. The sprawling South Acton Estate in Ealing was one of the largest in Britain and in need of urgent regeneration, with decaying properties and antisocial behaviour an ever-growing concern; the extent of the problem led to locals labelling the railway line dividing Chiswick and South Acton the 'Berlin Wall'. Acton Gardens is transforming these perceptions and the estate into a thriving mixed-tenure neighbourhood, replacing 1,800 obsolete and life-expired homes, which failed to meet residents' aspirations for modern homes standards, with 3,400 new homes between 2011 and 2029, and transforming life expectations.

The story

The approach of Countryside Partnerships to healthy placemaking is intrinsically related to sustainability, environmental quality and community cohesion. Successful, sustainable communities enjoy a sense of place and are diverse and inclusive. They encourage active involvement in their design and management through proper engagement and the nurturing of community spirit. They are connected, are walkable and have a wide range of social facilities. Designing for flexibility in future patterns of living and working is important. This is the 'Countryside Way'.

The objectives of the partnership (Countryside Partnerships, L&Q and Ealing Council) and masterplan design aims to integrate the new place into the surrounding areas, both physically and socially. This is achieved through the scale of the buildings, roads and walking routes, as well as the creation of new shops and parks that people from outside the estate want to visit, a GP surgery, dentist surgery and community centre that are used by all, a diverted bus route, and community development practices and investment that encourage social integration.

In order to ensure a socially sustainable future for the area, a genuinely mixed community is being created. The allows for 50 per cent affordable housing (with a mix of affordable rent and shared ownership) and 26 per cent family housing, along with the provision of new social infrastructure for local residents, including over 13,000 m² of public space, with new streets, parks and sports facilities.

Since 2011, 1,513 new homes have been built, with a further 412 under construction. The sales strategy has also had considerable success in targeting owner-occupiers. This is important to ensure the community can develop and sustain itself over time as the regeneration moves through the estate. The homes being delivered also include a range of design features to encourage sustainable living and reduce inhabitants' carbon footprint, such as green roofs, photovoltaic (PV) panels and combined heat and power (CHP) engines in a communal energy centre to supply the development's heat and power.

With 1,800 households, 24 community groups, two schools, churches, a community centre and various clubs in existence before the start of the project, and with the aim of breaking down the social boundaries that divided the old estate and neighbouring communities, community engagement could not be more important to Acton Gardens. To achieve this, four full-time members of staff located on site ensure effective communication through:

• a staffed regeneration and residents' liaison office;
• evening surgeries;
• a community board;
• a community chest;
• focus groups;
• website and newsletters;
• a housing management team;
• estate enhancement projects involving Cultivate London; and
• resident integration events, such as a summer party, outdoor cinema and BBQ.

Andrew takes three workstreams to illustrate Countryside Partnerships' approach.

The Acton Gardens Community Board

The Acton Gardens Community Board is the formal resident involvement structure between the residents of Acton Gardens and South Acton and the partnership of L&Q, Countryside Partnerships and Ealing Council. The Acton Gardens Community Board oversees the regeneration of South Acton by:

- providing feedback on the regeneration;
- ensuring that there is continued community involvement;
- encouraging participation from under-represented groups;
- allocating community chest funding for local projects; and
- attending tours, training, subgroups and consultation events for feedback.

Each year, £50,000 is made available for applications from local groups, with up to £5,000 being offered per project. To date, Countryside Partnerships have funded nearly 100 projects, including gardening, sports, education, music, community days, support groups and arts projects.

Cultivate London

As part of the regeneration, Countryside Partnerships are supporting Cultivate London in providing local unemployed people with 'work-ready' experience, landscaping and horticulture training, as well as other community-focused initiatives. Cultivate London is an innovative urban farm and social enterprise located across derelict sites in West London. They train unemployed young people in landscaping and horticulture, and produce edible and ornamental plants for sale.

The main aim is to have a long-term impact on the lives of young people and to change the way Londoners think about their fresh produce and where it comes from. The project has created a plant nursery on site, purchased plants to use in the landscaping areas and provided estate management and community events for the new community.

Research

Acton Gardens is going beyond other regeneration schemes by pioneering new methods to best measure the impact of the regeneration, demonstrating a genuine commitment to improving lives in the area. Independent analysts from the University of Reading and Social Life are measuring how the regeneration is improving lives, socially and economically, over the lifetime of the development. Monitoring the impact on society and the economy plays an important part in understanding, and, if necessary, altering, the approach to community development and support. Initial findings indicate that residents' perceptions of safety have improved, with people reporting higher levels of wellbeing and satisfaction.

Conclusion

The three parts of the project described are an integral part of the overall project to change and improve lives. Learning from estate regeneration also rings true for new communities and urban extensions. Involving the community in key decisions through the community board, providing skills, training and employment for local people, and conducting timely research to enable learning in real time are all vital to ensure that the new community not only delivers quality new homes, but also transforms life expectations.

Developers need to deliver more than just bricks and mortar; they need to build communities as well. The Acton Gardens project has demonstrated that through concerted effort and continual joint working with communities, developers can deliver meaningful change to lives and outcomes. The research has demonstrated real-time change occurring as a result of the regeneration and partnership working.

Further information

Further details of Countryside Partnerships and the Acton Gardens development are available at: www.countrysidepartnerships.com/all-developments/london/acton-gardens

Concluding reflections

> The data has shown a willingness on the part of the public to change and to adopt new healthy habits when required to. Spreading the practice of spatial planning public health across disciplines and sectors can help build a safer and more secure future for everyone.
>
> Outterside and Chang (2020)

The vision of the future was very different before the COVID-19 pandemic – and when the authors conceived the idea for this publication in early 2019. Its lasting effect, combined with accelerated and changing societal trends, has opened the door for a significant social and political discourse around the purpose of spatial planning that has, in turn, assembled complex scenarios to observe. At its very least, the COVID-19 pandemic has re-emphasised the need for good housing, access to green space, proximity to social and community infrastructure and services, and a healthy public realm.

Table C.1 brings together a range of factors that should be considered to help professionals identify and forecast the likelihood of occurrence and the degree of certainty that such trends will take place in the future, and the impacts these may have on public health. It can help professionals future-proof the policies they advocate and decisions they influence, and can be used as a tool to support prioritisation for actions.

Planning is a technical activity focusing on immediate consenting needs, as well as visionary strategic activity often looking 10–20-plus years into the future. If planning for health practitioners are to realise a vision of healthy and equitable places and communities, they must do better at foresight to

Table C.1: Public health spatial planning horizon-scanning matrix

Trends/factors	Likelihood of occurrence	Level of certainty	Global to local impact	Prioritisation for action
Societal and cultural				
Economic		PLACE		
Environmental				
Political	PEOPLE		PLANNING	
Technological				
Health		PUBLIC HEALTH		
Legal				

identify, discuss, discount or act as and when necessary. The following themes are the authors' attempt to start to identify some significant challenges and opportunities to be aware of for the future.

Deregulation

The ongoing challenges posed by deregulation and its impact on planning policies and resultant decisions that affect people's relationship with the environment will continue to underpin professional discourse in the foreseeable future. Policy and planning agendas are constantly evolving, particularly when they are partly influenced by changes to wider ideological discourse at the national and local levels.

There are competing threats and opportunities of deregulation versus a more interventionist, regulatory approach guiding planning processes. There are benefits to simplifying planning regulations for a variety of reasons, including streamlining the process to unclutter the system, improving accessibility by the public to strip out overcomplicated technical assessments and removing unnecessary burdens on businesses and system users to allow minor works to take place without a bureaucratic and expensive application process.

However, there are also threats and adverse effects that flow from deregulation and giving greater freedom to market forces, including removing the ability of local decision-makers to manage unwanted development, introducing new measures to speed up development without checks and balances on quality standards, and undermining established principles of public participation in the planning process. Strengthening, not weakening, the role and status of professionals to advise politicians and decision-makers on the costs and benefits of deregulation will become increasingly important.

Legacy impact from the pandemic

COVID-19 has raised the profile and national debate for how individuals, whole communities and places experience and interact with spaces and places in the public realm. For example, whether planning policy and practices are responding to changing high-street landscapes and a corresponding rise in online shopping and home deliveries (Deloitte, 2021) or additional space requirements in the new homeworking normal (Barratt Developments and Lichfields, 2021). The experience of the pandemic and the world slowly adjusting to it becoming an ongoing and endemic concern have put into focus the interrelated and localised impact that spatial planning policies and developments have on public health, and vice versa. Health protection and containment of the virus have been at the heart of most nations' responses to the pandemic (Green et al, 2020a, 2021b). Such impacts have been found to be distributed across society in an uneven way, impacting disadvantaged places and communities the most (Marmot et al, 2020b).

If communities, societies and governments are to 'build back better' or deliver on the 'levelling up' agenda, communities, governments and systems will have to deal with post-pandemic consequences. Therefore, adopting a place-making approach that supports HiAP and integrated working between public health and planning systems must be at the heart of decision-making. Public health spatial planning practitioners have an essential role to play in building healthy and equitable communities that are also more resilient to future pandemics.

Climate emergency

If the new kid on the block of health challenges is COVID-19, then the truculent teenager who is proving even more intractable to deal with effectively is the climate emergency. Climate change has been called the biggest global health threat of the 21st century (Watts et al, 2018). The world is at a critical juncture in relation to climate change, and extreme weather events are becoming increasingly common. Climate change has a major impact, both directly and indirectly, not only on the way that space and land are allocated and utilised, but also on how this will impact health and wellbeing, as well as pressures on healthcare infrastructure and services (PHW, 2021a; WHO, 2021a).

The public health sector and the health services serving communities will need to adapt, respond and become more resilient to climate challenges by supporting planners to shape a more sustainable environment. Unless we start designing and building in ways which are sustainable and support mitigation and adaptation to a changing climate, we will see an exponential effect on the quality of people's daily lives and the viability of our health systems being threatened. Similarly, planning policies must support individual and community-wide responses to adopt more sustainable lifestyles and to reduce carbon footprints, for example, through greater uptake of active travel, thinking about what we eat and how our food is produced, and by doing what we can to reduce, reuse and recycle waste.

Obesity and the environment

Obesity is a huge challenge and priority to be tackled. High levels of overweight and obesity across the world are complicated by wider issues of poverty, food supply, food insecurity and malnutrition in many other countries (United Nations, 2019). This is exacerbated by high levels of physical inactivity, partly as a result of poor provision of active travel options and the adoption of more sedentary lifestyles. The indirect impact must also be considered, for example, how healthy (or less healthy) food environments are permitted to locate in close proximity to, and be more prevalent in, certain communities, and how houses and services are configured to promote healthier lifestyles.

Having a positive policy framework for a healthier food environment is a 'win–win' for planning and public health authorities, businesses and, most importantly, consumers and communities – a key co-benefit of using an HiAP approach. A renewed focus of planning to build sustainable and high-quality places should also ensure that new less healthy food outlets are not approved where they will impact negatively on eating behaviours, ultimately contributing to obesity rates. Such a positive approach would allow certainty for businesses around expectations for healthier food provision when applying for planning permission, and businesses and consumers to benefit from a better, more diverse and healthier retail offer in their neighbourhoods. These are also key areas where those seeking further deregulation or more interventionist approaches may be played out.

Changing food consumption and access trends

Linked to the obesity issue, there are changing trends in the way people have greater and more convenient access to food, and how food companies are responding to exponentially increasing demand. Some of these trends have accelerated due to COVID-19, including an increase in home ordering for takeaway deliveries, which has been seen in many nations (Chang et al, 2020).

Out-of-home food-sales data for the UK collected during COVID-19 from takeaways and fast-food outlets show a 245 per cent year-on-year growth in spending on meal deliveries, and there has been substantial growth in takeaways and deliveries, with quick-service restaurant chains more profitable in 2020 than 2019. Increasing online delivery sales, with a greater number of options within the catchment area, will translate to increasing land-use implications for new stores and increasing physical presence in non-traditional locations outside the usual high street and neighbourhood centre. There is already evidence of the emergence of dark or ghost kitchens operated by online delivery companies in existing warehousing and industrial sites with greater reach to consumers.

Final book remarks

The preceding examples are but a select few planning and health challenges on the horizon. As we demonstrated earlier, similar arguments can be made for many other diseases affecting all societies, such as cardiovascular disease, many cancers or a variety of mental health and musculoskeletal conditions. The science of epidemiology and the art of public health spatial planning require practitioners to understand future trends and scenarios, and the evidence base for 'what works', and for the planning system to be fleet of foot when adapting and responding to new and evolving land-use activities.

The need for spatial planners and public health systems and practitioners to work together is becoming ever-more critical to avoiding the unintended negative consequences of policies and plans. Indeed, we believe that if we can succeed in the reunion of health and planning, we stand a good chance of making health improvement become a fundamental planning design principle to support the creation of healthy, environmentally sustainable, fair and prosperous communities for millions of people living in rural communities and urban areas alike. Planning for health will not happen by default, so there is a need to act now.

There were, there are and there will continue to be barriers, but these can and will be overcome. As we have demonstrated in this book, progress is being made in many areas within existing regulatory frameworks, for example, when national governments, public health institutions, public agencies, local authorities and local communities have proactively worked to make it happen. The extent of existing good practice already suggests that the ability to take action now is not a question of permissibility by law or policy, but one of political, professional, educational and practical willingness and confidence, or the lack thereof.

The authors began this book by setting out three propositions that formed a fundamental narrative shaping the development throughout:

- *The built and natural environments matter to health.* There are significant health inequalities between communities related, in part, to environmental hazards, the quality of the built environment and access to the natural environment. Early death and disability are the consequences for many of those living in such communities.

- *Planning matters to health.* A shared understanding and knowledge of the art and science of the possible by taking an HiAP approach and maximising the use of existing powers and tools can be applied to demonstrate the health gain to be achieved from policies and plans in a systematic and transparent manner, and to aid the decision-making process.
- *The professional workforce matters to health.* The public health spatial planning practitioner is a growing sub-specialism of both public health and planning that is on the rise. There is a need to learn from what is happening, to support institutional capacity building and to look afresh at professional training curricula to support building the current and future workforce.

The journey in the practice of public health spatial planning may be long for some and shorter for others. It is the sincere hope of the authors that this book helps to clear the path towards healthier, more equitable and fairer communities and environments.

Post-reading reflection

Now, having read this book, put the book down and go outside again or reflect on your day-to-day work practices. Retrace your steps. Notice your surroundings and how it might be impacting on your health. Then, note down what actions you are able to take individually or collectively at work to make the environment better for health and wellbeing. We look forward to you implementing your actions and reaping the benefits as a planning for health practitioner with important responsibilities and capabilities for making a difference.

APPENDIX

Practical resources

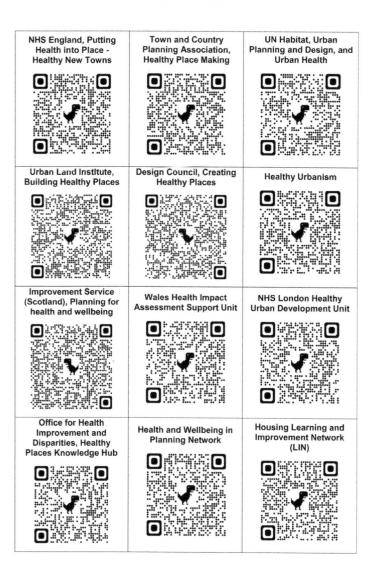

NHS England, Putting Health into Place - Healthy New Towns	Town and Country Planning Association, Healthy Place Making	UN Habitat, Urban Planning and Design, and Urban Health
Urban Land Institute, Building Healthy Places	Design Council, Creating Healthy Places	Healthy Urbanism
Improvement Service (Scotland), Planning for health and wellbeing	Wales Health Impact Assessment Support Unit	NHS London Healthy Urban Development Unit
Office for Health Improvement and Disparities, Healthy Places Knowledge Hub	Health and Wellbeing in Planning Network	Housing Learning and Improvement Network (LIN)

References

Adams D. (2021) 'Planning and development', in Parker G. and Street E. (eds) *Contemporary Planning Practice. Skills, Specialisms and Knowledge*, London: Red Globe Press, pp 91–105.

Aldred R. and Verlinghieri E. (2020) 'LTNs for all? Mapping the extent of London's new low traffic neighbourhoods', Active Travel Academy.

APSE (Association for Public Sector Excellence) (2020) 'At a crossroads. Building foundations for healthy communities'. Available from: www.apse.org.uk/apse/index.cfm/research/current-research-programme/at-a-crossroads-building-foundations-for-healthy-communities (accessed 21 May 2022).

Barratt Developments and Lichfields (2021) 'Working from home. Planning for the new normal?'. Available from: https://lichfields.uk/content/insights/working-from-home (accessed 1 January 2022).

Barton H. and Grant M. (2006) 'A health map for the local human habitat', *The Journal of the Royal Society for the Promotion of Health*, 126(6): 252–3.

Belfast Healthy Cities (2014) 'Reuniting planning and health. Planning healthy communities resource pack'. Available from: https://planning.belfasthealthycities.com/planning-healthy-communities-resource-pack (accessed 13 January 2021).

Benusic M. (2014) 'Health impact assessments are long overdue', *British Colombia Medical Journal*, 56(5): 238–39.

Bhavsar N.A., Kumar M. and Richman L. (2020) 'Defining gentrification for epidemiologic research: a systematic review', *PLoS ONE*, 15(5): e0233361.

Bird E.L., Ige J., Pilkington P., Pinto A., Petrokofsky C. and Burgess-Allen J. (2018) 'Built and natural environment planning principles for promoting health: An umbrella review', *BMC Public Health*, 18: 930.

Birley M.H. (2011) *Health Impact Assessment: Principles and Practice*, London: Earthscan.

Birley M.H., Boland A., Davies L., Edwards R.T., Glanville H., Ison E., Millstone E., Osborn D., ScottSamuel A. and Treweek J. (1998) *Health and Environmental Impact Assessment: An Integrated Approach*, London: Earthscan and British Medical Association.

Black D., Ayres S., Bondy K., Brierley R., Campbell R., Carhart N. et al (2021) 'Tackling root causes upstream of unhealthy urban development (TRUUD): protocol of a five-year prevention research consortium', *Wellcome Open Research*, 6: 30.

Blackshaw J. and van Dijk M. (2019) 'Health matters: whole systems approach to obesity'. Available from: https://publiche althmatters.blog.gov.uk/2019/07/25/health-matters-whole-systems-approach-to-obesity (accessed 21 January 2021).

Blanc F., Boyle J., Crook T., Scanlon K., Smith S. and Whitehead C. (2021) *The Value, Incidence and Impact of Developer Contributions in Scotland*, Edinburgh: Scottish Government.

Braveman, P. and Gottlieb, L. (2014) 'The social determinants of health: it's time to consider the causes of the causes', *Public Health Reports*, 129(Suppl 2): 19–31.

BRE (Building Research Establishment) (2018) *Home Quality Mark ONE. Technical Manual. England, Scotland and Wales*. Available from: www.homequalitymark.com/professionals/standard/ (accessed 21 May 2022).

BRE Academy (no date) 'Home Quality Mark training'. Available from: www.bre.co.uk/academy/hqm (accessed 5 April 2021).

Bristow A. (2021) 'Meeting the housing needs of BAME households in England: the role of the planning system'. Available from: https://i-sphere.site.hw.ac.uk/2021/08/23/role-of-planning-in-meeting-housing-needs-of-bame-hou seholds-in-england (accessed 20 December 2021).

British Columbia Centre for Disease Control (2019) *Healthy Built Environment Linkages Toolkit: Making the Links between Design, Planning and Health, Version 2.0*, Vancouver, BC: Provincial Health Services Authority.

Brown J.A., Gorman M., Kim H.J., Schober K., Vipond J. and Nykiforuk C. (2020) 'Scoping population health in impact assessment (ScopHIA) realist review: identifying best practices for equity in scoping of major natural resource and large-scale infrastructure projects', research report for the 'Informing Best Practices for Environmental and Impact Assessments' Knowledge Synthesis Grants competition launched by the Social Sciences and Humanities Council of Canada and Impact Assessment Agency of Canada, School of Public Health, University of Alberta.

Building Better, Building Beautiful Commission (2019) *Creating Space for Beauty the Interim Report of the Building Better, Building Beautiful Commission.* Available from: www.gov.uk/governm ent/groups/building-better-building-beautiful-commission (accessed 21 May 2022).

Cabinet Office (2009) *The Wider Costs of Transport in English Urban Areas in 2009,* London: Cabinet Office Strategy Unit.

Campbell Collaboration (2022) 'Campbell's vision, mission and key principles'. Available from: www.campbellcollaborat ion.org/about-campbell/vision-mission-and-principle.html (accessed 8 January 2022).

Carmichael L. and Richmond C. (2020) 'Health impact assessment. Policy in the London Borough of Tower Hamlets', *Impact Assessment Outlook Journal – Health Impact Assessment in Planning. Thought Pieces from UK Practice,* 8: 8–10.

Carmichael L., Townshend T., Fischer T. and Lock, K (2019) 'Urban planning as an enabler of urban health: challenges and good practice in England following the 2012 planning and public health reforms', *Land Use Policy,* 84: 154–62.

Cave B., Ison E., Pyper R., Reeves A., Azam S. and Green L. (2016) *Health in All Policies. All Policies in Health,* Leeds: Ben Cave Associates on behalf of Public Health Wales.

Cave B., Fothergill J., Pyper R., Gibson G. and Saunders P. (2017) *Health in Environmental Impact Assessment: A Primer for a Proportionate Approach,* London: IEMA.

Cave B., Claßen T., Fischer-Bonde B., Humboldt-Dachroeden S., Martín-Olmedo P., Mekel O., Pyper R., Silva F., Viliani F. and Xiao Y. (2020) 'Summary of human health: ensuring a high level of protection. A reference paper on addressing human health in environmental impact assessment as per EU Directive 2011/92/EU amended by 2014/52/EU'. North Dakota: International Association for Impact Assessment and European Public Health Association.

Cave B., Pyper R., Fischer-Bonde B., Humboldt-Dachroeden S. and Martin-Olmedo P. (2021) 'Lessons from an international initiative to set and share good practice on human health in environmental impact assessment', *International Journal of Environmental Research and Public Health*, 18(4): 1392.

Cavill N., Davis A., Cope A. and Corner D. (2019) *Active Travel and Physical Activity Evidence Review*, London: Sport England.

Center for Active Design (2020) 'Reference guide for the Fitwel certification system: community (beta), version 2.1'. Available from: www.fitwel.org/resources (accessed 15 December 2021).

Center for Active Design (2021) *A New Investor Consensus: The Rising Demand for Healthy Buildings. Health and Real Estate Investment Survey Results*, BentallGreenOak, the Center for Active Design and United Nations Environment Programme Finance Initiative (UNEP FI).

Chadderton C., Elliott E., Hacking N., Shepherd M. and Williams G. (2013) 'Health impact assessment in the UK planning system: the possibilities and limits of community engagement', *Health Promotion International*, 28(4): 533–43.

Chang M. (2017) 'Who pays and who benefits? Understanding the value of investing in "healthy places"', *Town & Country Planning*, May: 187–92.

Chang M. and Radley D. (2020) 'Using planning powers to promote healthy weight environments in England', *Emerald Open Research*, 2: 68.

Chang M. and Ross A. (2012) 'Reuniting health with planning', *Town & Country Planning*, 81: 307–8.

Chang M., Green L. and Cummins S. (2020) 'All change. Has COVID-19 transformed the way we need to plan for a healthier and more equitable food environment?', *Urban Design International*, 26: 291–5.

Chilaka M.A. (2010) 'Vital statistics relating to the practice of health impact assessment (HIA) in the United Kingdom', *Environmental Impact Assessment Review*, 30(2): 116–19.

CIPD (Chartered Institute of Personnel and Development) (2020) 'Workforce planning'. Available from: www.cipd.co.uk/knowledge/strategy/organisational-development/workforce-planning-factsheet#gref (accessed 4 April 2021).

Cochrane A.L. (1972) *Effectiveness and Efficiency: Random Reflections on Health Services*, London: Nuffield Trust.

Cochrane Collaboration (2022) 'Homepage'. Available from: www.cochrane.org

Cooke A. and Stansfield J. (2009) *Improving Mental Well-Being through Impact Assessment (NMHDU): A Summary of the Development and Application of a Mental Well-Being Impact Assessment Tool*, London: National Mental Health Development Unit.

Cooke A., Friedli L., Coggins T., Edmonds N., Michaelson J., O'Hara K., Snowden L., Stansfield J., Steuer N. and Scott-Samuel A. (2011) *Mental Wellbeing Impact Assessment. A Toolkit for Wellbeing* (3rd edn), London: National MWIA Collaborative.

Croal P., Tetreault C. and members of the International Association for Impact Assessment Indigenous Peoples Section (2012) *Respecting Indigenous Peoples and Traditional Knowledge*, Special Publication Series No. 9, Fargo, ND: International Association for Impact Assessment.

Crook T., Henneberry J., Rowley S., Watkins C. and Wells J. (2006) *Valuing Planning Obligations in England*, London: DCLG.

Dahlgren G. and Whitehead M. (2007) 'Policies and strategies to promote social equity in health. Background document to WHO – strategy paper for Europe', Arbetsrapport, 2007:14, Institute for Futures Studies.

Dannenberg L., Frumkin H. and Jackson R. (eds) (2011) *Making Healthy Places. Designing and Building for Health, Well-Being and Sustainability*, Washington, DC: Island Press.

DCLG (2012) 'National Planning Policy Framework'. Available from: www.gov.uk/guidance/national-planning-policy-framework (accessed 1 July 2021).

DCLG (2016) 'Government response to the report of the House of Lords Select Committee on the Built Environment presented to Parliament by the Secretary of State for Communities and Local Government by Command of Her Majesty'. London: DCLG.

Defra (Department for Environment, Food and Rural Affairs) (2012) 'Biodiversity offsetting pilots technical paper: the metric for the biodiversity offsetting pilot in England'. London: Defra.

Defra (2018) *A Green Future: Our 25 Year Plan to Improve the Environment*, London: Defra.

Delany T., Lawless A., Baum F., Popay J., Jones L., McDermott D., Harris E., Broderick D. and Marmot M. (2016) 'Health in All Policies in South Australia: what has supported early implementation?', *Health Promotion International*, 31(4): 888–98.

Deloitte (2021) 'What next for the high street?'. Available from: www2.deloitte.com/uk/en/pages/consumer-business/articles/what-next-for-the-high-street.html (accessed 11 January 2022).

Department of Health (2011) *Joint Strategic Needs Assessment and Joint Health and Wellbeing Strategies Explained: Commissioning for Populations*, London: Department of Health.

Department of Health (2013) *Health Building Note 00–09: Infection Control in the Built Environment*, London: Department of Health.

DHSC (2021) 'Public health ring-fenced grant 2021 to 2022: local authority circular'. Available from: www.gov.uk/government/publications/public-health-grants-to-local-authorities-2021-to-2022/public-health-ring-fenced-grant-2021-to-2022-local-authority-circular (accessed 1 May 2021).

Douglas M. (2019) *Health Impact Assessment Guidance for Practitioners*, Edinburgh: Scottish Health and Inequalities Impact Assessment Network and Scottish Public Health Network.

ECHP (European Centre for Health Policy) (1999) 'Gothenburg consensus paper – health impact assessment: main concepts and suggested approach', European Centre for Health Policy.

Edmonds N., Parry-Williams L. and Green L. (2019) *WHIASU Training and Capacity Building Framework for HIA in Wales*, Wrexham: WHIASU.

Egan Review (2004) *The Egan Review: Skills for Sustainable Communities*, London: Office of the Deputy Prime Minister.

Elliott E. and Williams G. (2008) 'Developing public sociology through health impact assessment', *Sociology of Health & Illness*, 30(7): 1101–16.

EuroHealthNet (2019) 'Health Inequalities in Europe'. Available from: https://eurohealthnet.eu/wp-content/uploads/docume nts/2019/191023_Factsheet_HealthEquityEU_WebLayout.pdf (accessed 15 January 2022).

European Parliament and Council of the European Union (2001) 'Directive 2001/42/EC of the European Parliament and of the Council on the assessment of the effects of certain plans and programmes on the environment', *Official Journal of the European Communities*. Available from: http://data.europa. eu/eli/dir/2001/42/oj (accessed 6 June 2021).

European Parliament and Council of the European Union (2014) 'Directive 2014/52/EU of the European Parliament and of the Council of 16 April 2014 amending Directive 2011/92/EU on the assessment of the effects of certain public and private projects on the environment text with EEA relevance', L 124/ 1. Available from: http://eur-lex.europa.eu/legal-content/ EN/TXT/PDF/?uri=CELEX:32014L0052&from=EN (accessed 6 June 2021).

Evans K. and Boyce K. (2008) 'Fostering a hierarchy of evidence within the profession', *Journal of Diagnostic Medical Sonography*, 24: 183–8.

Fischer T.B. (2007) *Theory and Practice of Strategic Environmental Assessment*, London: Earthscan.

Fischer T.B. and Cave B. (2018) 'Health in impact assessments – introduction to a special issue', *Impact Assessment and Project Appraisal*, 36(1): 1–4.

Fischer T.B., Mulhoora, T. and Smith M. (2020) 'Links between health issues and the development of strategic plans'. Available from: www.pas.gov.uk/pas/plan-making/strategic-plans/ strategic-planning-research-paper-links-between-health-iss ues-and#6conclusions-and-recommendations (accessed 1 February 2021).

FPH (Faculty of Public Health) (2016) 'Good public health practice framework'. Available from: www.fph.org.uk/profe ssional-development/good-public-health-practice (accessed 1 February 2021).

FPH (2020) 'Continuing professional development (CPD) policies, processes and strategic direction'. Available from: www.fph.org.uk/media/1435/cpd-policy-from-1-april-2014-updated-july-2016.pdf (accessed 21 May 2022).

Frank L.D., Kershaw S.E., Chapman J.E. and Perrotta K. (2014) *Residential Preferences and Public Health in Metro Vancouver: Promoting Health and Well Being by Meeting the Demand for Walkable Urban Environments*, Vancouver: Health and Community Design Lab, University of British Columbia.

Fredsgaard M.W., Cave B. and Bond A. (2009) *A Review Package for Health Impact Assessment Reports of Development Projects*, Leeds: Ben Cave Associates.

Freiler A., Muntaner C., Shankardass K., Mah C.L., Molnar A., Renahy E. and O'Campo P. (2013) 'Glossary for the implementation of Health in All Policies (HiAP)', *Journal of Epidemiology and Community Health*, 67(12): 1068–72.

Garrett H., Mackay M., Nicol S., Piddington J. and Roys, M. (2021) *The Cost of Poor Housing to the NHS: 2021 Briefing Paper*, Watford: BRE Trust.

Geddes I., Allen J., Allen M. and Morrisey L. (2011) *The Marmot Review: Implications for Spatial Planning*, London: National Institute for Health and Care Excellence (NICE).

Geertse M. (2008) 'Garden cities to the world! The international propagation of the garden city idea 1913–1926', paper presented at the 7th European Social Science History conference, Lisbon University, Portugal.

Glazener A., Sanchez K., Ramani T., Zietsman J., Nieuwenhuijsen M.J., Mindell J.S., Fox M. and Khreis H. (2021) 'Fourteen pathways between urban transportation and health: a conceptual model and literature review', *Journal of Transport & Health*, 21.

Government of Canada (2019) 'Impact Assessment Act 2019'. Available from: https://laws.justice.gc.ca/eng/acts/I-2.75/index.html (accessed 21 May 2022).

Green L., Parry-Williams L. and Edmonds N. (2017) *Quality Assurance Review Framework for Health Impact Assessment (HIA)*, Wrexham: WHIASU.

Green L., Gray B.J., Edmonds N. and Parry-Williams L. (2019) 'Development of a quality assurance review framework for health impact assessments', *Impact Assessment and Project Appraisal*, 37(2): 107–13.

Green L., Morgan L., Azam S., Evans L., Parry-Williams L., Petchey L. and Bellis M.A. (2020a) *A Health Impact Assessment of the 'Staying at Home and Social Distancing Policy' in Wales in Response to the COVID-19 Pandemic. Main Report*, Cardiff: Public Health Wales.

Green L., Lewis R., Evans L., Morgan L., Parry-Williams L., Azam S. and Bellis M.A. (2020b) *A COVID-19 Pandemic World and Beyond: The Public Health Impact of Home and Agile Working in Wales. Summary Report*, Cardiff: Public Health Wales NHS Trust.

Green L., Gray B. and Ashton K. (2020c) 'Using health impact assessments to implement the Sustainable Development Goals in practice: a case study in Wales', *Impact Assessment and Project Appraisal*, 38(3): 214–24.

Green L., Ashton K., Edmonds N. and Azam S. (2020d) 'Process, practice and progress: a case study of the health impact assessment (HIA) of Brexit in Wales', *International Journal of Environmental Research and Public Health*, 17(18): 6652.

Green L., Parry-Williams L. and Huckle E. (2021a) *Health Impact Assessment (HIA) and Local Development Plans (LDPs): A Toolkit for Practice*, Cardiff: Public Health Wales.

Green L., Ashton K., Azam S., Dyakova M., Clements T. and Bellis M.A. (2021b) 'Using health impact assessment (HIA) to understand the wider health and wellbeing implications of policy decisions: the COVID-19 "staying at home and social distancing policy" in Wales', *BMC Public Health*.

Griffiths, H. (2021) 'The high cost of low traffic neighbourhoods', *Auto Express*, 26 January. Available from: www.autoexpress.co.uk/low-traffic-neighbourhoods (accessed 16 January 2022).

Haigh F., Harris E., Harris-Roxas B., Baum F., Dannenberg A.L., Harris M.F. et al (2015) 'What makes health impact assessments successful? Factors contributing to effectiveness in Australia and New Zealand', *BMC Public Health*, 1009: 1–2.

Harris P., Harris-Roxas B., Harris E. and Kemp L. (2007) 'Health impact assessment: a practical guide', Centre for Health Equity Training, Research and Evaluation (CHETRE), UNSW Research Centre for Primary Health Care and Equity, UNSW.

Harris P., Sainsbury P. and Kemp L. (2014) 'The fit between health impact assessment and public policy: practice meets theory', *Social Science and Medicine*, 108: 46–53.

Harris-Roxas A.B. and Harris P.J. (2007) 'Learning by doing: the value of case studies of health impact assessment', *New South Wales Public Health Bulletin*, 18: 161–3.

Health Foundation (2018) 'What makes us healthy? An introduction to the social determinants of health'. Available from: www.health.org.uk/publications/what-makes-us-heal thy (accessed 1 June 2021).

Health Foundation (2021) 'Frequency of active travel by local authority'. Available from: www.health.org.uk/evidence-hub/ transport/active-travel/frequency-of-active-travel-by-local-authority (accessed 1 May 2021).

Health Knowledge (2021) 'Concepts of health and well-being'. Available from: www.healthknowledge.org.uk/public-hea lth-textbook/medical-sociology-policy-economics/4a-conce pts-health-illness/section2/activity3

Higgins J.P.T., Thomas J., Chandler J., Cumpston M., Li T., Page M.J. and Welch V.A. (eds) (2021) 'Cochrane handbook for systematic reviews of interventions', version 6.2, February. Available from: www.training.cochrane.org/handbook (accessed 8 January 2022).

HMSO (Her Majesty's Stationery Office) (2013) 'Explanatory memorandum to the Community Infrastructure Levy (Amendment) Regulations 2013'. Available from: www.legislat ion.gov.uk/uksi/2013/982/memorandum/contents (accessed 22 May 2022).

Horizon Nuclear Power (2018) 'Wylfa Newydd Project. 8.18 Health impact assessment non-technical summary'. Available from: https://infrastructure.planninginspectorate.gov.uk/wp-content/ipc/uploads/projects/EN010007/EN010007-001 737-8.18%20Health%20Impact%20Assessment%20Non-Technical%20Summary%20(Rev%201.0).pdf (accessed 8 January 2022).

House of Commons Health Select Committee (2015) *Childhood Obesity – Brave and Bold Action. First Report of Session 2015–16*, London: The Stationery Office.

House of Commons Health Select Committee (2018) *Childhood Obesity: Time for Action*, London: The Stationery Office.

House of Lords (2016) *House of Lords Select Committee on National Policy for the Built Environment. Report of Session 2015–16. Building Better Places*, London: The Stationery Office.

Huang Z. (2012) 'Health impact assessment in China: emergence, progress and challenges', *Environmental Impact Assessment Review*, 32(1): 45–9.

Hunter D. (2017) 'Policy-makers' hierarchy of evidence: adapted from Davies (2005) with acknowledgements to Hunter, D; *Health in All Policies: Making it Work in Practice*', Winter School, Durham University.

Hunter R.F., Cleland C., Cleary A., Droomers M., Wheelerd B.W., Sinnett D., Nieuwenhuijsen M.J. and Braubach M. (2019) 'Environmental, health, wellbeing, social and equity effects of urban green space interventions: a meta-narrative evidence synthesis', *Environment International*, 130: 2–20.

Ige J., Pilkington P., Orme J., Williams B., Prestwood E., Black D., Carmichael L. and Scally G. (2019) 'The relationship between buildings and health: a systematic review', *Journal of Public Health*, 41(2): e121–32.

Ige J., Pilkington P., Bird E., Gray S., Mindell J., Chang M., Stimpson A., Gallagher D. and Petrokofsky C. (2020) 'Exploring the views of planners and public health practitioners on integrating health evidence into spatial planning in England: a mixed-methods study', *Journal of Public Health*, 10: 1093.

IWBI (International WELL Building Institute) (2020) 'WELL v2'. Available from: https://v2.wellcertified.com/wellv2/en/overview (accessed 5 April 2021).

Johnson T. and Green L. (2021) 'Planning and enabling healthy environments'. Available from: https://whiasu.publichealth network.cymru/en/resources?cat=3&keyword=&topics= (accessed 1 June 2021).

Keeble M., Burgoine T., White M., Summerbell C., Cummins S. and Adams J. (2019) 'How does local government use the planning system to regulate hot food takeaway outlets? A census of current practice in England using document review', *Health & Place*, 57: 171–8.

Kemm J. (2003) 'Perspectives on health impact assessment', *Bulletin of the World Health Organisation*, 81(6): 387.

Kemm J., Parry, J. and Palmer, S. (eds) (2004) *Health Impact Assessment: Concepts, Theory, Techniques and Applications*, Oxford: Oxford University Press.

Kögel C.C., Rodríguez Peña T., Sánchez I., Tobella M., López J.A., Espot F.G., Claramunt F.P., Rabal G. and González Viana A. (2020) 'Health impact assessment (HIA) of a fluvial environment recovery project in a medium-sized Spanish town', *International Journal of Environmental Research and Public Health*, 17(5): 1484.

Landscape Institute (2020) 'Landscape Institute entry standards and competency framework – core landscape competencies'. Available from: www.landscapeinstitute.org/education/intr oducing-the-new-entry-standards-and-competency-framew ork (accessed 21 January 2021).

Lanktree, G. (2019) 'The great Section 106 and CIL scandal', *Property Week*, 27 September. Available from: www.propertyw eek.com/insight/the-great-section-106-and-cil-scandal/5104 449.article (accessed 1 May 2021).

Larson J.S. (1999) 'The conceptualization of health', *Medical Care Research and Review*, 56(2): 123–36.

Leppo K., Ollila E., Peña S., Wismar M. and Cook S. (eds) (2013) *Health in All Policies: Seizing Opportunities, Implementing Policies*, Helsinki: Ministry of Social Affairs and Health of Finland.

LGA (Local Government Association) (2016) *Health in All Policies: A Manual for Local Government*, London: LGA.

LGA (2018a) *Childhood Obesity Trailblazer Programme. Prospectus*, London: LGA.

LGA (2018b) *Public Health Transformation Five Years on Transformation in Action*, London: LGA.

Lichfields (2018a) 'Solutions to an age old problem. Planning for an ageing population'. Available from: https://lichfields.uk/content/insights/solutions-to-an-age-old-problem (accessed 5 April 2021).

Lichfields (2018b) 'Local choices? Housing delivery through neighbourhood plans'. Available from: https://lichfields.uk/media/4128/local-choices_housing-delivery-through-neighbourhood-plans.pdf (accessed 5 April 2021).

Littell J. and White H. (2018) 'The Campbell Collaboration: providing better evidence for a better world', *Research on Social Work Practice*, 28(1): 6–12.

Lord A., Dunning R., Buck M., Cantillon S., Burgess G., Crook T., Watkins C. and Whitehead C. (2020) *The Incidence, Value and Delivery of Planning Obligations and Community Infrastructure Levy in England in 2018–19*, London: MHCLG.

Macfadyen N. (2013) *Health and Garden Cities. A Re-Publication of the Garden Cities and Town Planning Association Pamphlet on the Health Benefits of Garden Cities* (Town & Country Planning, Tomorrow Series, Paper 14), London: TCPA.

Mahoney M.E., Potter J.L. and Marsh R.S. (2007) 'Community participation in HIA: discords in teleology and terminology', *Critical Public Health*, 17(3): 229–41.

Marmot M., Allen J., Goldblatt P., Boyce T., McNeish D. and Grady M. (2010) *Fair Society, Healthy Lives: The Marmot Review*, London: Institute of Health Equity.

Marmot M., Allen J., Boyce T., Goldblatt P. and Morrison J. (2020a) *Health Equity in England: The Marmot Review 10 Years On*, London: Institute of Health Equity.

Marmot M., Allen J., Goldblatt P., Herd E. and Morrison J. (2020b) *Build Back Fairer: The COVID-19 Marmot Review. The Pandemic, Socioeconomic and Health Inequalities in England*, London: Institute of Health Equity.

Marselle M.R., Bowler D.E., Watzema J., Eichenberg D., Toralf K. and Bonn A. (2020) 'Urban street tree biodiversity and antidepressant prescriptions', *Scientific Reports*, 10: 22445.

Marsh R., Chang M. and Wood J. (2020) 'The relationship between housing created through permitted development'. *Cities & Health*, DOI: 10.1080/23748834.2020.1833281

Marteau T., Rutter H. and Marmot M. (2021) 'Changing behaviour: an essential component of tackling health inequalities', *BMJ*, 372. doi:10.1136/bmj.n332

Maula A., LaFond N., Orton E., Iliffe S., Audsley S., Vedhara K. and Kendrick D. (2019) 'Use it or lose it: a qualitative study of the maintenance of physical activity in older adults', *BMC Geriatrics*, 19: 349.

McGill E., Egan M., Petticrew M. et al (2015) 'Trading quality for relevance: non-health decision-makers' use of evidence on the social determinants of health', *BMJ Open*, 5: e007053.

McGowan V.J., Buckner S., Mead R., McGill E., Ronzi S., Beyer F. and Bambra C. (2021) 'Examining the effectiveness of place-based interventions to improve public health and reduce health inequalities: an umbrella review', *BMC Public Health*, 21: 1888.

McKeown T. and Lowe C.R. (1974) *An Introduction to Social Medicine* (2nd edn), Oxford: Blackwell Scientific Publications.

McKinnon G., Pineo H., Chang M., Taylor-Green L., Jones A. and Toms R. (2020) 'Strengthening the links between planning and health in England', *BMJ*. Available from: www.bmj.com/content/369/bmj.m795 (accessed 10 May 2021).

McQueen D., Wismar M., Lin V., Jones C. and Davies M. (2012) 'Intersectoral governance for Health in All Policies. Structures, actions and experiences', World Health Organization on behalf of the European Observatory on Health Systems and Policies.

MHCLG (Ministry of Housing, Communities and Local Government) (2019) 'Planning practice guidance. Planning obligations'. Available from: www.gov.uk/guidance/planning-obligations (accessed 30 April 2021).

MHCLG (2020) *English Housing Survey 2019 to 2020: Headline Report*, London: MHCLG.

MHCLG (2021a) 'Message from the Chief Planner', *Planning Newsletter*, No. 1, 5 February. Available from: https://assets.publishing.service.gov.uk/government/uploads/system/uploads/attachment_data/file/959245/Chief_Planners_Newsletter_-_February_2021.pdf (accessed 1 June 2021).

MHCLG (2021b) *National Planning Policy Framework*, London: MHCLG.

MHCLG (2021c) *National Design Guide*, London: MHCLG.

MHCLG (2021d) *National Model Design Code*, London: MHCLG.

Mindell J., Biddulph J., Taylor L., Lock K., Boaz A., Joffe M. and Curtis S. (2010) 'Improving the use of evidence in health impact assessment', *Bulletin of the World Health Organization*, 88(7): 543–50.

Moore T.H.M., Kesten J.M., López-López J.A., Ijaz S., McAleenan A., Richards A., Gray S., Savović J. and Audrey S. (2018) 'The effects of changes to the built environment on the mental health and well-being of adults: systematic review', *Health Place*, 53: 237–57.

Morgan R.K. (2011) 'Health and impact assessment: are we seeing closer integration?', *Environmental Impact Assessment Review*, 31(4): 404–11.

Morley R., Sambunjak D., Watts C. and Morley K. (2019) 'Module 1: Evidence-based medicine', in Cochrane (ed) *Cochrane Evidence Essentials*. Available from: https://training.cochrane.org/essentials (accessed 30 April 2021).

Mundo W., Manetta P., Fort M. and Sauaia A. (2019) 'A qualitative study of health in all policies at the local level', *Journal of Health Care Organization*, Provision, and Financing, 5 September.

Natural England (2021) 'Introduction to the green infrastructure framework – principles and standards for England'. Available from: https://designatedsites.naturalengland.org.uk/GreenInfrastructure/Home.aspx (accessed 15 January 2022).

Nau T., Smith B.J., Bauman A. and Bellew B. (2021) 'Legal strategies to improve physical activity in populations' ['Stratégies juridiques d'amélioration de l'activité physique au sein des populations'], *Bulletin of the World Health Organization*, 99(8): 593–602.

NHS Digital (2018) 'Health survey for England'. Available from: https://digital.nhs.uk/data-and-information/publications/statistical/health-survey-for-england/2018/summary (accessed 15 January 2022).

NHS Digital (2019) 'Statistics on obesity, physical activity and diet, England'. Available from: https://digital.nhs.uk/data-and-information/publications/statistical/statistics-on-obes ity-physical-activity-and-diet/statistics-on-obesity-physical-activity-and-diet-england-2019/part-5-adult-physical-activity (accessed 15 January 2022).

NHS England (2019) 'Putting health into place. Principles 1–3. Plan, assess and involve'. Available from: www.england.nhs. uk/ourwork/innovation/healthy-new-towns/ (accessed 10 January 2022).

Nieuwenhuijsen M.J. (2016) 'Urban and transport planning, environmental exposures and health – new concepts, methods and tools to improve health in cities', *Environmental Health*, 15: S38.

Nottinghamshire County Council (2019) 'Nottinghamshire spatial planning and health framework 2019–2022'. Available from: www.nottinghamshire.gov.uk/planning-and-environm ent/planning-and-health-framework/planning-and-health-framework-2019-2022 (accessed 20 December 2021).

Núñez-González S., Delgado-Ron J.A., Gault C., Lara-Vinueza A., Calle-Celi D., Porreca R. and Simancas-Racines D. (2020) 'Overview of "systematic reviews" of the built environment's effects on mental health', *Journal of Environmental and Public Health*, 19: 9523127.

Nutbeam, D. (2020) 'Developing health public policy', in I. Kawachi, I. Lang and W. Ricciardi (eds) *The Oxford Handbook of Public Health Practice*, Oxford: Oxford University Press, pp 304–311.

O'Malley, C.L., Lake, A.A., Townshend, T.G. and Moore, H.J. (2021) 'Exploring the fast food and planning appeals system in England and Wales: decisions made by the Planning Inspectorate (PINS)', *Perspectives in Public Health*, 141(5): 269–278.

ONS (Office for National Statistics) (2019) 'Urban green spaces raise nearby house prices by an average of £2,500'. Available from: www.ons.gov.uk/economy/environmentalaccounts/ articles/urbangreenspacesraisenearbyhousepricesbyanaverag eof2500/2019-10-14 (accessed 30 May 2021).

ONS (2021) 'How has lockdown changed our relationship with nature?'. Available from: www.ons.gov.uk/economy/enviro nmentalaccounts/articles/howhaslockdownchangedourrelatio nshipwithnature/2021-04-26 (accessed 30 May 2021).

Outterside A. and Chang M. (2020) 'The pandemic and positive lifestyle changes', *Transforming Society*. Available from: www.tran sformingsociety.co.uk/2020/09/04/the-pandemic-and-posit ive-lifestyle-changes (accessed 11 May 2021).

Parry J. and Scully E. (2003) 'Health impact assessment and the consideration of health inequalities', *Journal of Public Health*, 25(3): 243–5.

Parry J. and Stevens A. (2001) 'Prospective health impact assessment: pitfalls, problems, and possible ways forward', *BMJ (Clinical Research Edn)*, 323(7322): 1177–82.

PHE (Public Health England) (2014) 'Everybody active every day: an evidence based approach to physical activity'. Available from: https://assets.publishing.service.gov.uk/government/ uploads/system/uploads/attachment_data/file/374914/Frame work_13.pdf (accessed 16 January 2022).

PHE (2016) *Working Together to Promote Active Travel: A Briefing for Local Authorities*, London: PHE.

PHE (2017) *Spatial Planning for Health: An Evidence Resource for Planning and Designing Healthier Places*, London: Public Health England.

PHE (2018) *Healthy High Streets*, London: PHE.

PHE (2019a) 'Physical activity: applying all our health'. Available from: www.gov.uk/government/publications/physical-activ ity-applying-all-our-health/physical-activity-applying-all-our-health (accessed 8 September 2021).

PHE (2019b) *Review of Interventions to Improve Outdoor Air Quality and Public Health*, London: PHE.

PHE (2020a) 'Case study. Town planning and public health: shared competencies'. Available from: www.gov.uk/gov ernment/case-studies/town-planning-and-public-health-sha red-competencies?utm_medium=email&utm_source=govd elivery (accessed 15 January 2021).

PHE (2020b) *Health Impact Assessment in Spatial Planning: A Guide for Local Authority Public Health and Planning Teams*, London: PHE.

PHE (2020c) *Improving Access to Greenspace a New Review for 2020*, London: PHE.

PHE (2020d) 'Health matters: physical activity – prevention and management of long-term conditions'. Available from: www. gov.uk/government/publications/health-matters-physical-activity/health-matters-physical-activity-prevention-and-man agement-of-long-term-conditions#wider-role-and-benefits-of-physical-activity (accessed 16 January 2022).

PHE (2021) 'Health profile for England'. Available from: https:// fingertips.phe.org.uk/static-reports/health-profile-for-engl and/hpfe_report.html#summary-11---healthy-life-expecta ncy (accessed 15 January 2022).

PHW (2021a) 'Health and wellbeing impacts of climate change'. Available from: https://phw.nhs.wales/news/new-resou rce-highlights-health-impacts-of-climate-change (accessed 2 February 2022).

PHW (2021b) 'Mental wellbeing impact assessment'. Available from: www.publichealthnetwork.cymru/en/topics/health-imp act-assessment/mental-wellbeing-impact-assessment (accessed 1 June 2021).

Pineo H., Glonti K., Rutter H., Zimmermann N., Wilkinson P. and Davies M. (2018) 'Urban health indicator tools of the physical environment: a systematic review', *Journal of Urban Health*, 95: 613–46.

Pineo H., Thrift J. and Chang M. (2021) 'Planning for health and well-being', in Parker G. and Street E. (eds) *Contemporary Planning Practice. Skills, Specialisms and Knowledge*, London: Red Globe Press.

Place Alliance (2020) 'A housing design audit for England'. Available from: https://placealliance.org.uk/research/natio nal-housing-audit/ (accessed 18 January 2022).

POST (Parliamentary Office of Science and Technology) (2014) *POSTNOTE 458. Ambient Air Quality*, London: Houses of Parliament.

Prüss-Ustün A., Wolf J., Corvalán C., Bos R. and Neira M. (2016) *Preventing Disease Through Healthy Environments: A Global Assessment of the Burden of Disease from Environmental Risks*, Geneva: WHO.

Public Health Scotland (2017) 'The Place Standard tool'. Available from: www.healthscotland.scot/health-inequalities/impact-of-social-and-physical-environments/place/the-place-standard-tool (accessed 1 June 2021).

Public Health Scotland (2021) 'Place and wellbeing: integrating land use planning and public health in Scotland' Available from: www.improvementservice.org.uk/products-and-servi ces/consultancy-and-support/planning-for-place-programme/ place-health-and-wellbeing (accessed 22 May 2022).

Pyper R., Cave B., Purdy J. and McAvoy, H. (2021) *Health Impact Assessment Guidance: A Manual. Standalone Health Impact Assessment and Health in Environmental Assessment*, Dublin and Belfast: Institute of Public Health.

Ramirez-Rubio O., Daher C., Fanjul G., Fanjul G., Gascon M., Mueller N., Pajín L., Plasencia A., Rojas-Rueda D., Thondoo M. and Nieuwenhuijsen M.J. (2019) 'Urban health: an example of a "Health in All Policies" approach in the context of SDGs implementation', *Global Health*, 15(1): 87.

Rao M., Prasad S., Adshead F. and Tissera H. (2007) 'The built environment and health', *The Lancet*, 370(9593): 1111–13.

RCEP (Royal Commission on Environmental Pollution) (2007) *The Urban Environment*, London: TSO.

RICS (Royal Institution for Chartered Surveyors) (2012) *Financial Viability in Planning. RICS Guidance Note* (1st edn), London: RICS.

RICS (2016) *RICS Professional Guidance, UK Placemaking and Value* (1st edn), London: RICS.

Roger Tym & Partners (2010) 'Training in development economics: Equipping the planning sector with skills to manage deliverability and viability'. London: Roger Tym & Partners.

Rogerson B., Lindberg R., Baum F., Dora C., Haigh F., Simoncelli A., Parry-Williams L., Peralta G., Pollack P., Keshia M. and Solar O. (2020) 'Recent advances in health impact assessment and Health in All Policies implementation: lessons from an international convening in Barcelona', *International Journal of Environmental Research and Public Health*, 17(21): 7714.

Rojas-Rueda D., Nieuwenhuijsen M.J., Gascon M., Perez-Leon D. and Mudu P. (2019) 'Green spaces and mortality: a systematic review and meta-analysis of cohort studies', *The Lancet Planetary Health*, 3(11): e469–77.

Rosenberg W. and Donald A. (1995) 'Evidence based medicine: an approach to clinical problem-solving', *BMJ*, 310(1): 122–6.

Ross, A. and Chang, M. (2012) *Reuniting Health with Planning*, London: TCPA.

Rowley S., Crook T., Henneberry J. and Watkins C. (2007) 'The use and value of planning obligations in Wales. A report to the Welsh Assembly Government'. Available from: https://gov.wales/use-and-value-planning-obligations (accessed 7 December 2021).

RPS Group (2015) 'Hinkley Point C health impact assessment'. Available from: https://infrastructure.planninginspectorate.gov.uk/wp-content/uploads/2010/01/Hinkley-Point-C-EIA-Scoping-Report.pdf (accessed 1 June 2021).

RTPI (Royal Town Planning Institute) (2014) *Promoting Healthy Cities – Why Planning Is Critical to a Healthy Urban Future*, London: RTPI.

RTPI (2017) 'Ethics and professional standards. Advice for RTPI members'. Available from: www.rtpi.org.uk/membership/professional-standards/professional-ethics (accessed 21 January 2021).

RTPI (2020) 'Enabling healthy placemaking. Overcoming barriers and learning from best practices', RTPI Research Paper. Available from: www.rtpi.org.uk/healthyplacemaking (accessed 21 January 2021).

Scarborough P., Bhatnagar P., Wickramasinghe KK., Allender S., Foster C. and Rayner M. (2011) 'The economic burden of ill health due to diet, physical inactivity, smoking, alcohol and obesity in the UK: an update to 2006–07 NHS costs', *Journal of Public Health*, 33(4): 527–35.

Scottish Government (2013) 'Strategic environment assessment: guidance'. Available from: www.gov.scot/publications/strategic-environmental-assessment-guidance/ (accessed 6 June 2021).

Scottish Government (2020) 'Planning obligations and good neighbour agreements (revised November 2020)', Circular 3/2012.

Shankardass K., Renahy E., Muntaner C. and O'Campo P. (2015) 'Strengthening the implementation of Health in All Policies: a methodology for realist explanatory case studies', *Health Policy and Planning*, 30(4): 462–73.

Shankardass K., Muntaner C., Kokkinen L., Shahidi F.V., Freiler A., Oneka G., Bayoumi A. and O'Campo P. (2018) 'The implementation of Health in All Policies initiatives: a systems framework for government action', *Health Research Policy and Systems*, 16(1): 26.

Sharpe C.A., Chang M., Petrokofsky C. and Stimpson A. (2021) 'Health impact assessment in spatial planning in England', *Cities & Health*, DOI: 10.1080/23748834.2021.1876377.

Simpson S., Mahoney M., Harris E., Aldrich R. and Stewart-Williams J. (2005) 'Equity-focused health impact assessment: a tool to assist policy makers in addressing health inequalities', *Environmental Impact Assessment Review*, 25(7–8): 772–82.

SOPHIA (Society of Practitioners of Health Impact Assessment) (2021) 'HIA guidance and tools'. Available from: www.hiasoci ety.org (accessed 6 June 2021).

Ståhl T. (2018) 'Health in All Policies: from rhetoric to implementation and evaluation – the Finnish experience', *Scandinavian Journal of Public Health*, 46(20_suppl): 38–46.

Stappers N.E.H., Van Kann D.H.H., Ettema D., De Vries N.K. and Kremers S.P.J. (2018) 'The effect of infrastructural changes in the built environment on physical activity, active transportation and sedentary behavior – a systematic review', *Health and Place*, 53: 135–49.

Stokes J. 3rd, Noren J. and Shindell S. (1982) 'Definition of terms and concepts applicable to clinical preventive medicine', *Journal of Community Health*, 8(1): 33–41.

Stringer v Minister of Housing and Local Government (1970) 1 WLR 1281. Available from: http://www.hwa.uk.com/site/wp-content/uploads/2018/02/CD.CAS_.8-Stringer-v.-Minister-of-Housing-and-Local-Government-1971-1-All-ER-651.pdf (Accessed 14 July 2022).

Sustain (2019) 'Hot food takeaways: planning a route to healthier communities'. Available from: www.sustainweb.org/publications/hot_food_takeaways/ (accessed 1 March 2021).

Sustrans (no date) 'What is a low traffic neighbourhood'. Available from: www.sustrans.org.uk/our-blog/get-active/2020/in-your-community/what-is-a-low-traffic-neighbourhood (accessed 30 May 2021).

Tajima R. and Fischer T.B. (2013) 'Should different impact assessment instruments be integrated? Evidence from English spatial planning', *Environmental Impact Assessment Review*, 41: 29–37.

Tamburrini A., Gilhuly K. and Harris-Roxas B. (2011) 'Enhancing benefits in health impact assessment through stakeholder consultation', *Impact Assessment and Project Appraisal*, 29(3): 195–204.

Tamm M.E. (1993) 'Models of health and disease', *British Journal of Medical Psychology*, 66(3): 213–28.

TCPA (Town and Country Planning Association) (2012) *Reuniting Health with Planning – Healthier Homes, Healthier Communities*, London: TCPA.

TCPA (2015) *Public Health in Planning. Good Practice Guide*, London: TCPA.

TCPA (2017) 'The Raynsford review of planning. Creating a blueprint for a new planning system. Background paper 2: the rise and fall of town planning'. Available from: www.tcpa.org.uk/raynsford-review (accessed 14 January 2021).

TCPA (2018) *Securing Constructive Collaboration and Consensus for Planning Healthy Developments: A Report from the Developers and Wellbeing Project*, London: TCPA.

TCPA (2019) 'The state of the union. Reuniting health with planning in promoting healthy communities'. Available from: www.rtpi.org.uk/healthyplacemaking (accessed 21 January 2021).

TCPA and WHIASU (Wales Health Impact Assessment Support Unit) (2016) *Planning for Better Health and Well-Being in Wales: A Briefing on Integrating Planning and Public Health for Practitioners Working in Local Planning Authorities and Health Organisations in Wales*, Wrexham: WHIASU.

Tcymbal A., Demetriou Y., Kelso A., Wolbring L., Wunsch K., Wäsche H. et al (2020) 'Effects of the built environment on physical activity: a systematic review of longitudinal studies taking sex/gender into account', *Environmental Health and Preventive Medicine*, 25: 75.

Therival R. (2010) *Strategic Environmental Assessment in Action* (2nd edition). London: Earthscan.

Therival R. and Partido M.R. (2013) *The Practice of Strategic Environmental Assessment*, Abingdon: Routledge.

Thomas C., Round A. and Longlands S. (2020) *Levelling Up Health for Prosperity*, London: Institute for Public Policy Research.

Townshend, T. (2022) *Healthy Cities? Design for Well-Being*, London: Lund Humphries.

Transport for All (2021) 'Pave the way'. Available from: www.transportforall.org.uk/wp-content/uploads/2021/01/Pave-The-Way-full-report.pdf (accessed 30 May 2021).

Transport for West Midlands (2018) '*Movement for Growth*, health and transport strategy'. Available from: www.tfwm.org.uk/who-we-are/our-strategy/movement-for-growth-strategic-transport-plan/ (accessed 16 Jan 2022).

Turnbull R. (2021) 'Healthy, happy places – a more integrated approach to creating health and well-being through the built environment?', *British Medical Bulletin*, 140: 62–75.

UK Built Environment Advisory Group (2018) 'Commonwealth built environment professionals commit to working more effectively "towards a common future"'. Available from: www.architecture.com/about/uk-built-environment-advisory-group (accessed 19 April 2021).

UKCMO (UK Chief Medical Officers) (2019) *UK Chief Medical Officers' Physical Activity Guidelines*, London: UK Department of Health and Social Care, Llwodraeth Cymru Welsh Government, Department of Health Northern Ireland, and the Scottish Government.

UKGBC (UK Green Building Council) (2020) *Driving Social Value in New Development: Options for Local Authorities*, London: UKGBC.

Ulrich R. (1984) 'View through a window may influence recovery from surgery', *Science*, 224(4647): 420–1.

UNECE (United Nations Economic Commission for Europe) (2015) *Convention on Environmental Impact Assessment in a Transboundary Context. Adopted in Espoo (Finland), on 25 February 1991 as amended on 27 February 2001*, Geneva: UNECE.

UNECE (2019) *Draft Guidance on Assessing Health Impacts in Strategic Environmental Assessment (SEA)*, Geneva: UNECE.

UN-Habitat and World Health Organization (2020) 'Integrating health in urban and territorial planning: a sourcebook'. Available from: https://unhabitat.org/sites/default/files/2020/05/1-final_highres_20002_integrating_health_in_urban_and_territorial_planning_a_sourcebook.pdf

United Nations (1992) 'Report of the United Nations Conference on Environment and Development', Rio de Janeiro, 3–14 June.

United Nations (2019) *The State of Food Security and Nutrition in the World. Safeguarding against Economic Slowdowns and Downturns*, Rome: Food and Agriculture Organization of the United Nations.

United Nations Environment (2018) *Assessing Environmental Impacts: A Global Review of the Evidence*, Kenya: UNE.

University of Ottawa (2021) 'Definitions of health'. Available from: www.med.uottawa.ca/courses/CMED6203/Index_notes/Definitions%20of%20Health.htm (accessed 19 April 2021).

Urban Land Institute (2021) *Zooming in on the 'S' in ESG: A Road Map for Social Value in Real Estate*, London: Urban Land Institute.

Van Eyk H., Harris E., Baum F., Delany-Crowe T., Lawless A. and MacDougall C. (2017) 'Health in All Policies in South Australia – did it promote and enact an equity perspective?', *International Journal of Environmental Research and Public Health*, 14(11): 1288.

Vanclay F. (2003) 'International principles for social impact assessment', *Impact Assessment and Project Appraisal*, 21(1): 5–11.

Walker G., Fairburn J., Smith G. and Mitchell G. (2003) *Environmental Quality and Social Deprivation* (R&D Technical Report E2-067/1/TR), Bristol: Environment Agency.

Watts N. Amann M., Arnell N., Ayeb-Karlsson S., Belesova K., Berry H. et al (2018) 'The 2018 report of the Lancet Countdown on health and climate change: shaping the health of nations for centuries to come', *The Lancet*, 392(10163): 2479–514.

Wells N., Evans G. and Yang Y. (2010) 'Environments and health: planning decisions as public-health decisions', *Journal of Architectural and Planning Research*, 27(2): 124–43.

Welsh Government (2020) 'Local development plan manual (edition 3) consultation document'. Available from: https://gov.wales/development-plans-manual-edition-3-march-2020 (accessed 27 May 2021).

Welsh Government (2021a) 'Planning policy Wales, edition 11'. Available from: https://gov.wales/sites/default/files/publi cations/2021-02/planning-policy-wales-edition-11_0.pdf (accessed 27 May 2021).

Welsh Government (2021b) 'Future Wales integrated sustainability appraisal'. Available from: https://gov.wales/fut ure-wales-integrated-sustainability-appraisal-non-technical-summary (accessed 27 May 2021).

WHIASU (Wales Health Impact Assessment Support Unit) (2012) *Health Impact Assessment. A Practical Guide*, Wrexham: WHIASU.

WHIASU (2021) 'Population group checklists'. Available from: https://whiasu.publichealthnetwork.cymru/en/resour ces/ (accessed 8 December 2020).

White J.T., Kenny T., Samuel F., Foye C., James G. and Bilge S. (2020) *Delivering Design Value: The Housing Design Quality Conundrum*, Glasgow: UK Collaborative Centre for Housing Evidence.

WHO (1946) 'Constitution of the World Health Organisation'. Available from: www.who.int/about/who-we-are/constitution (accessed 1 June 2021).

WHO (1986) 'Ottawa Charter for Health Promotion'.

WHO (2010a) 'Health impact assessment: decisions and policy making'. Available from: www.who.int/news-room/q-a-det ail/health-impact-assessment-decisions-and-policy-making (accessed 1 June 2021).

WHO (2010b) *Adelaide Statement on Health in All Policies: Moving Towards a Shared Governance for Health and Well-Being*, Adelaide, South Australia: World Health Organization and Government of South Australia. Available from: www.who.int/social_d eterminants/publications/isa/hiap_statement_who_sa_final. pdf?ua=1 (accessed 1 June 2021).

WHO (2013a) *Global Action Plan for the Prevention and Control of Noncommunicable Disease 2013–2020*, Geneva: WHO.

WHO (2013b) *Health 2020. A European Policy Framework and Strategy for the 21st Century*, Geneva: WHO.

WHO (2014) 'Health in All Policies: Helsinki statement. Framework for country action'. Available from: www.who.int/publications/i/item/health-in-all-policies-helsinki-statem ent (accessed 8 December, 2020).

WHO (2015) *Health in All Policies: Training Manual*, Geneva: WHO.

WHO (2018a) *Key Learning on Health in All Policies Implementation from Around the World – Information Brochure*, Geneva: WHO.

WHO (2018b) *Physical Activity Factsheets for the 28 European Union Member States of the WHO European Region*, Geneva: WHO.

WHO (2019) *Urban Green Spaces: A Brief for Action*, Geneva: WHO.

WHO (2020a) 'Social determinants of health'. Available from: www.who.int/health-topics/social-determinants-of-hea lth#tab=tab_1 (accessed 1 June 2021).

WHO (2020b) 'Factsheets on physical activity'. Available from: www.who.int/news-room/fact-sheets/detail/physical-activity (accessed 29 May 2021).

WHO (2021a) 'Climate change and health'. Available from: www.who.int/news-room/fact-sheets/detail/climate-change-and-health (accessed 2 September 2021).

WHO (2021b) 'Health impact assessment'. Available from: www.who.int/health-topics/health-impact-assessment#tab=tab_1 (accessed 1 June 2021).

WHO (2021c) *Heat and Health in the WHO European Region: Updated Evidence for Effective Prevention*, Geneva: WHO.

WHO (2022) 'WHO European NCD dashboard'. Available from: www.euro.who.int/en/health-topics/noncommunica ble-diseases/pages/who-european-office-for-the-prevent ion-and-control-of-noncommunicable-diseases-ncd-office/ data-publications-and-tools/who-european-ncd-dashboard (accessed 5 February 2022).

Winkler M.S., Krieger G.R., Divall M.H., Cisse G., Wielga M., Singer B.H., Tanner M. and Utzinger J. (2013) 'Untapped potential of health impact assessment', *Bulletin of the World Health Organisation*, 91(4): 298–305.

Winkler M.S., Furu P., Viliani F., Cave B., Divall M., Ramesh G., Harris-Roxas B. and Knoblauch A.M. (2020) 'Current global health impact assessment practice', *International Journal of Environmental Research and Public Health*, 17(9): 2988.

Winkler M.S., Viliani F., Knoblauch A.M., Cave B., Divall M., Ramesh G., Harris-Roxas B. and Furu P. (2021) *Health Impact Assessment International Best Practice Principles* (Special Publication Series No. 5), Fargo, ND: International Association of Impact Assessment.

Wismar M., Blau J., Ernst K. and Figueras J. (eds) (2007) *The Effectiveness of Health Impact Assessment. Scope and Limitations of Supporting Decision-Making in Europe*, Geneva: World Health Organization on behalf of the European Observatory on Health Systems and Policy.

WMCA (West Midlands Combined Authority) (2016) *Movement for Growth: The West Midlands Strategic Transport Plan*, West Midlands Combined Authority. Available from: www.tfwm. org.uk/who-we-are/our-strategy/movement-for-growth-strategic-transport-plan/ (accessed 21 May 2022).

Woodbury G. and Kuhnke J. (2014) 'Evidence-based practice vs. evidence-informed practice: what's the difference?', *Wound Care Canada*, 12(1): 26–9.

Index

References to figures appear in *italic* type; those in **bold** type refer to tables.